CLICK IT TO RIP IT

BY
ANNA PETRAS CPT

CONTENTS

FOREWORD

G'day Ladies!

I'm Anna Petras, personal trainer and writer of your personal fitness guide, *Click it to Rip it*. Originally from Australia, my brother, sisters, and I grew up just 45 minutes from the beach in Brisbane and Melbourne. It's a lovely place filled with wonderful people, tropical birds, and, yes, kangaroos! I lived in Australia for much of my life, until my family and I were bit with the travel bug just over 12 years ago. We said "goodbye" to the outback and "hello" to the United States! With the exception of a few visits back to Australia, we've been in the U.S. ever since, in which time our family has grown. I am now an aunt to four boys and four girls, and spoiling them is one of my favorite hobbies.

One way I like to spoil my nieces and nephews is with delicious food, something of which I have developed a very different mentality over the years. Growing up, I never had to worry about what I ate, because I was always tiny and didn't gain any weight. However, in my early 20's, my body decided to turn on me. I was living in Florida and becoming acutely aware of my weight gain. It took 22 pounds of excess before I finally decided I had to make a change. For me, the realization hit suddenly, as though I woke up one morning and realized that I was overweight, that I felt sluggish all the time, and that I just didn't feel like my old self any more.I was far less flexible than I once was, and I simply didn't feel my absolute best. So, I wanted to make a change for myself.

Change is never easy, and my body was no exception. First, I tried all the easy ways out: alleged ab miracles I spotted on infomercials, strange diet pills, and various crash diets. As you might expect, none of these worked. Each time I gained back the auxiliary weight I'd lost, my spirit was crushed. But not destroyed. I was still determined, and I still pushed forward.

As a last resort, I turned to a gym and a personal trainer. At first, I was anxious—I was completely misinformed about how exercise can change your body and didn't expect to see results. But something incredible happened. After just 14 days of clean eating combined with a full body workout and cardio, I lost 15 pounds! I felt like a completely new person, and I was inspired to keep going.

This was the beginning of my new, fit and healthy lifestyle. Shortly after those two weeks, I had to quit working out with my trainer, and I couldn't keep my gym membership— I just couldn't afford it. So, I continued my new lifestyle at home, incorporating clean meals, a full body workout, and cardio three to four times a week.

My journey didn't end there, though. I became a Certified Personal Trainer, pursuing my newfound love and dream.

It became my mission to share my success and let every woman know that losing weight is not impossible. In fact, it can be fun and easy, especially with a little bit of guidance and support. So, I began training women from the comforts of their own homes, aiding in a long line of new success stories and newfound happiness.

In my training, I have found that every journey is unique, containing its own set of challenges. For me, my challenges came a few years ago. In 2011, I was experiencing major stomach pain, stomach distension, bloating, and cramping. My digestive system was less than normal, and when my pain reached a level that was simply unbearable, I decided to see a gastrologist. The gastrologist diagnosed me with IBS or Irritable Bowel Syndrome and suggested some prescription drugs as treatment. I didn't want to treat my symptoms with medication, so I worked to discover the cause. In discovering mild food allergies and sensitivities, I reworked my diet again and found incredible relief!

Once again, I was able to start a new life for myself. Ever since I began my fitness journey 9 years ago, my weight has stayed off. My body feels cleaner, lighter, and healthier than ever before, and it remains my mission to help every woman feel this way.

I have put together a full body workout plan for women who juggle many roles and obstacles. Because every life is filled with different challenges and obstacles, my plan acknowledges this and works around *your* schedule. I hope that you enjoy what I've put together for you. May it inspire and incite positive change in your life.

Cheers!

Anna Petras
Certified Personal Trainer

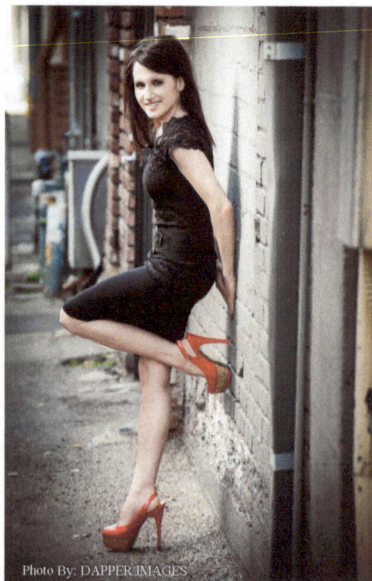

Photo By: DAPPER IMAGES

INTRODUCTION

Click it to Rip it[1] is your new personal fitness training guide! Each page is only a click away from a healthier, happier you and is filled with great tips for getting and staying in shape. The simplicity of the information makes it easy for you to follow, and the benefits you'll gain are HUGE. Throughout your fitness journey with *Click it to Rip it*, you will gain a great deal of knowledge while losing a great deal of excess fat and inches. Here's a little bit of what you'll learn:

- ☐ How to train your body

- ☐ How to stay healthy and fit when you travel

- ☐ How to maintain a healthy lifestyle, even if you're super busy

- ☐ How to cook and eat nutrient rich foods that are both tasty and healthy

- ☐ Important fitness facts that everyone should (but doesn't always) know

- ☐ What works best for you through a plethora of tips to keep you healthy and happy

☐ How to stay motivated so that you reach your weight loss and fitness goals!

The greatest part about all of these new insights is that you'll be able to do everything from the comfort of your own home. You can feel great without busting your budget on a gym membership and without wasting the extra time it takes to get to the gym.

Being fit and living a healthy lifestyle is something anyone can accomplish. My mission is to get this information into the hands of every woman who wants to make a change—to be in the best shape she can be and to feel *great* in her own skin!

Why *Click it to Rip it*?

I've said to myself, "Anna, you're a busy woman. But it's not impossible for you to be the best you can be."

With my time restraints, it just wasn't possible for me to go to the gym, but for me, being my best possible self meant staying healthy and fit. For years now, I've been active, working out 3-4 days a week; and I have sustained a healthy, fit lifestyle.

It is my goal to make my years of fitness knowledge public. I want women to know just how simple these lifestyle changes can be, and through *Click it to Rip it*, this shared knowledge is possible.

Via app and eBook, your personal fitness journey can be convenient, accessible, and simple. Just click it!

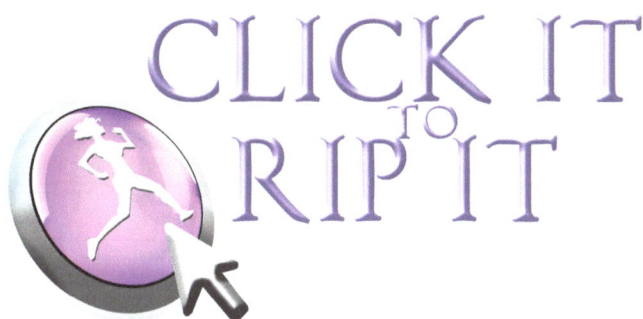

Click it to Rip it – **Full Body Workout App**

Our bodies are fascinating, and it's really important to keep our muscles challenged. How do we do this? By changing up our workout routine. The *Click it to Rip it©* app is wonderfully compatible with the eBook, because as you understand the body through reading, you can also experience the body with simple, step-by-step daily workout routines. All the workouts available are in constant rotation, so every day can hold a new challenge for both the mind and body.

The app includes two workout options. One is a workout using simple equipment (dumbbells and a stability ball). The other is without equipment, using your own body for resistance. Using simple tools like the dumbbells and the stability ball can amp up your routine greatly without incorporating equipment too complex or expensive for a home workout. Having a step-by-step, full body workout *without* equipment is great for the woman on the go. With both options conveniently in hand, you are guaranteed a daily guide for a full body workout, any place, any time.

Why *Click it to Rip it* Works for Women

Men's and women's bodies differ. Being a woman myself and training my own body, I tend to feel that my health and fitness expertise lies in the female body. However, women's bodies can differ greatly in shape even from one another (i.e. apple, pear, hourglass, ruler, etc.), giving us a wide range of "problem areas" and routine possibilities. This is why I've chosen to limit *Click it to Rip it* strictly to women. As you may have discovered, most workout programs are cookie-cutter or "universal," even though you and your body are unique. *Click it to Rip it* is designed to give you the knowledge and understanding of how to train YOUR BODY.

You may be thinking, "How intense is this program?" Don't worry…*Click it to Rip it* is not designed to break your back. *Click it to Rip it* is designed for a sustainable level of fitness. You may have found yourself drawn in by some intense programs out there that can give you fast results. However, it can be extremely difficult and dangerous to maintain this level of intensity. My workout programs will give you lasting results *without* the backbreaking intensity found in other programs.

Ladies, *Click it to Rip it* is easy to follow and easy to use.

INTRODUCTION

All it takes is dedication and time on your part. If you're serious about living a healthy lifestyle and dropping those extra pounds once and for all, *Click it to Rip it* will be with you every step of the way!

Click it to Rip it will help you get into the best shape possible with the full body workouts made especially for a woman's body—made especially for you! You have nothing to lose but the weight on your body. Plus, get ready to GAIN self-confidence and self-esteem, a healthy attitude towards your body and yourself, and personal power. When you look good, you feel good, and when you feel good, you radiate!

For your best results, I recommend working out at least 3-4 days a week. When you combine your workouts with a clean diet, you'll begin to see results within two weeks. You'll be motivated and thrilled with your results. All it takes is a little discipline and hard work and the belief that YOU CAN lose weight and feel great!

Sit back (for now) and get ready to *Click it to Rip it!*

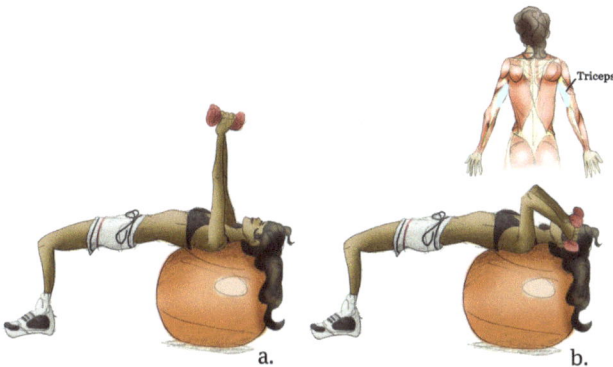

FIRST STEPS TO HEALTH AND HAPPINESS

I AM HERE TO HELP GUIDE YOU, but at the end of the day, this is *your journey! You* have the final say as to whether or not you're going to live a healthy, fit lifestyle, which can be both empowering and exciting! Here are some methods that worked for me and can work for you too:

1. The power of your own voice

Your words are powerful, and we are going to give them power by hearing them out loud. This is going to feel silly at first, but this method is extremely effective. I want you to say aloud to yourself...right now, "I promise that from this day forward, I commit to getting healthy and losing weight. I promise this to myself!"

Ok, because I *know* that you didn't really say it out loud, we'll count that silent reading as a practice round. This is for you, ladies! I want you to hear the power of your own voice and to make this powerful commitment *to yourselves*. All together now: *"I promise that from this day forward, I commit to getting healthy and losing weight! I promise this TO MYSELF!!"*

Wow, I'm really glad that you decided to shout that last part...it's a really important part of this mantra.

Now, I want you to write this affirmation on a piece of paper and stick it to your bathroom mirror. Every time you need a little encouragement, find it in *yourself*. Speak this mantra aloud to yourself as many times as necessary, and you will find all the encouragement you need.

2. The power of observing your thoughts

Henry Ford is famous in part for his quote: "Whether you think you can, or you think you can't--you're right."

This step, just like the first step, is to help you mentally prepare. Your mind is a powerful tool that can make or break your commitment to weight loss and getting healthy. Napoleon Hill, one of the leaders of the 'new thought movement' and author of *Think and Grow Rich* said, "The starting point of all achievement is DESIRE. Keep this constantly in mind. Weak desire brings weak results, just as a small fire makes a small amount of heat."

Give yourself some time now to self-reflect. What desires have made this weight creep onto your body throughout the past months and years? Maybe your desire was to have a baby (or maybe your desire led you to having a baby), and you now want to lose the baby weight. Maybe your desire lies in sweets, or maybe your desire comes from something that traces back to your childhood. Observe your thoughts as they come, not getting attached to any one thought.

Allow this process to continue until your mind is clear and calm. This may take a bit of time, and it may not all happen in one day. But your mental health is extremely important to your physical health. Now is the time for your healing from whatever it is that's been weighing you down, and now is the time to let go.

Your willpower, inner voice, and positive desires are what will ultimately drive you to health and happiness. Today, you allow your desire to be fit and healthy to overpower your desires to eat junk food, watch TV, sit on the computer—you name it. You are the ruler of your mind, and your desire to be healthy is most important. Today, your inner voice says, "I *am* worth it, and I *can* do this!"

3. The power of writing it down

Observing your thoughts is only one of many ways to self-reflect. You may also find it helpful to buy a journal or notebook and write down your thoughts. NO EDITING! Purge your mind until you can't write anymore. Get all of your thoughts and emotions out of your mind and body. Don't be afraid to let it all out in words *and tears*. Healing can be an emotional process, and that's okay. If you feel like you could cry for *hours*, cry for hours! This is healthy. Allowing yourself to feel your emotions, rather than finding the refuge you may have once found in food is both healthy and effective. Once you let out everything that's been re-pressed, bottled up, and forgotten, you are well on your way to your personal healing. You may be surprised at how letting out profound sadness can actually result in profound happiness! Not everyone is going to feel profoundly sad, of course, and that's good. But whatever it is you feel, don't be afraid to feel it! Once you've allowed yourself to face your fears and feelings, allow yourself to feel inspired!

4. The power of throwing it away

The next step is a kitchen makeover. I'm not talking new cabinets, new countertops, or even new doorknobs. This is a different kind of makeover.

Now is the time to clean out your cupboards, refrigerators, freezers, and pantries. Everything that screams junk food is to be tossed into the garbage. I know what you're thinking, "Food waste is terrible! Not to mention, I'm throwing away so much money!" The truth is, this food is not serving you, which means that it won't serve anybody! From now on, you are making a commitment to *yourself* to buy nutrient rich foods, which means that in the future, all the foods you donate or share with others will benefit *them* too!

By getting the junk food out of the house, you are releasing yourself from the temptation to eat unhealthy foods. Let's face it, when we're hungry, we want the quickest, easiest solution to our hunger. Unfortunately, those quick, easy solutions tend to be all of that *junk food!* And when we eat foods that are not nutrient rich, we eat empty calories and end up having to eat (and buy) *more* in order to feel satisfied. Now, you won't be tempted to munch on the bag of greasy chips or inhale a carton of your favorite ice cream

4

if they're no longer in your pantry or freezer. And that old junk drawer you had? Is now free for the taking!

When your pantry is clean, you feel much cleaner. When you eat cleanly, your insides feel the way that your new pantry makes you feel—flippin' amazing!

Go ahead…get on with your amazing self! I'll still be here when you get back.

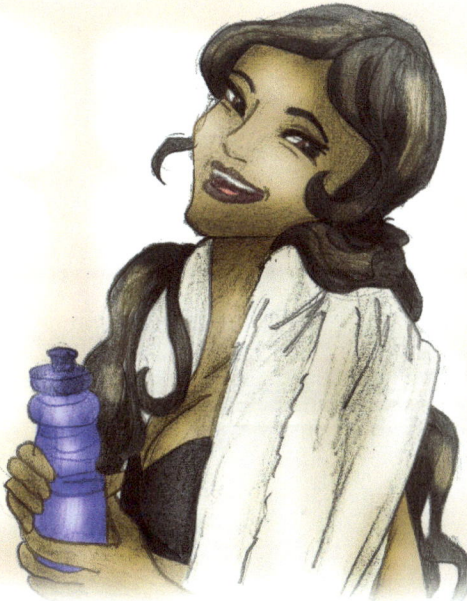

FULL BODY WORKOUT

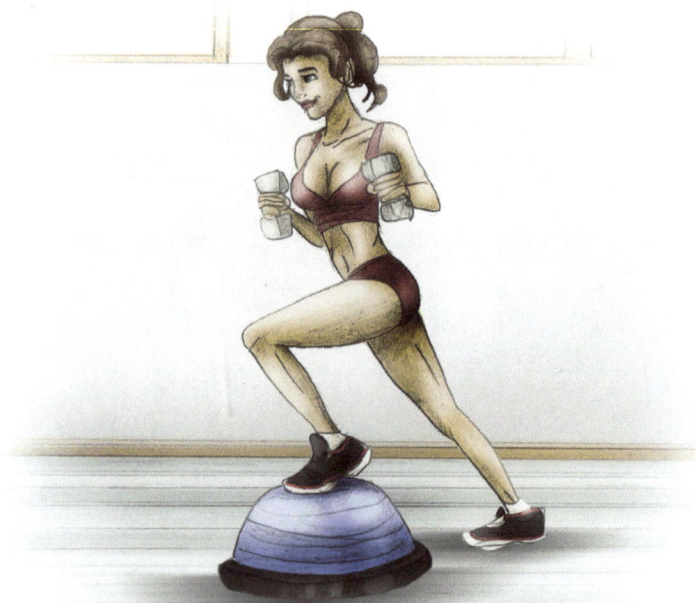

LADIES, IT'S TIME FOR YOU to get up and move your body. After all, if you want to lose 10 pounds, 15 pounds, 20 pounds, 30 pounds, or more than 50 pounds, you must move your body. It's time to stop making excuses for why you can't work out. We've all heard (and said) them before:

☐ I'm too tired.

☐ I don't have time to exercise.

☐ It will take too long for me to lose weight.

☐ It's too late for me to lose weight.

☐ What's the point?

☐ I'm too embarrassed to buy workout clothes.

☐ I'm too embarrassed to walk or run around the neighborhood.

☐ I don't know how to exercise.

☐ I can't do it.

Phew! Now that we've gotten that off our chests, it's time to kick these and other excuses to the curb and embrace the fact that YOU CAN work out and lose weight! The first thing you need to do is to shift your mindset. We're going to replace that negative tape that's been playing inside your head with a positive one. You are good enough! You are worth it! The fact that you're here right now means you've already taken the first and hardest step. You should be proud of yourself!

You may run into obstacles along the way, and that's okay! Get excited about facing these challenges and making these changes for yourself! Some obstacles can be very simply overcome. For instance, keep in mind that those who are not supportive are likely not supportive of themselves and should be paid no mind. You're losing weight for YOU, and that's a good enough reason for anybody. And even though your fitness journey is mainly for your own benefit, you will find all those around you benefitting as well (even the skeptics).

When you feel good in your own skin, you radiate, and your energy is infectious! If you have kids, you'll have more energy to play with them. If you're married or dating, you'll feel sexy and won't think twice about wearing that slinky black dress. You'll look forward to going to the doctor for your annual checkup, because you'll be in tip-top shape. The list is endless.

Working Out Safely

You should speak with your doctor before you begin any workout program, because he or she knows your medical history and will be able to help monitor your progress. Part of your doctor's job is also to promote a healthy lifestyle, so he or she is sure to be a great motivator. Your doctor might also have some workout tips and tricks of his or her own to share! Keep up with regular visits to your doctor to get personalized information about doing a workout plan that's safe and right for you.

The full body workout is your ticket to freedom:

☐ Freedom from this excess weight that's been weighing you down for too long

☐ Freedom to feel good about yourself

☐ Freedom to feel comfortable in your own skin

☐ Freedom to love, respect, and be grateful for your body.

Top Ten Benefits[2] of a Full Body Workout

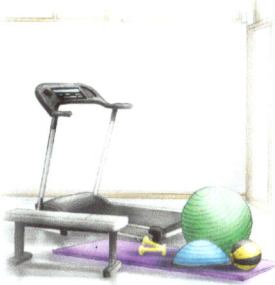

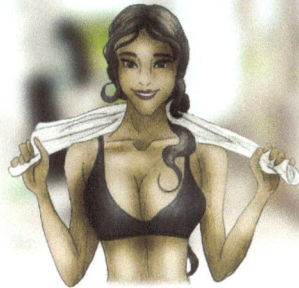

If you're pressed for time, a full body workout makes sense. You can work your arms, legs, abs, hips, buttocks, thighs, etc. all at once versus focusing on one area at a time.

Benefit #1 – Time restraint and commitment is lower

Most women are too busy to get to the gym, let alone to work out certain muscle groups on different days. A full body workout takes the stress out of working out because you work a number of your muscles all at once. There's no need to focus on abs one day and your arms the next. With a full body workout, your entire body is exercised at the same time. How efficient is that?

Benefit #2 – Greater muscle recovery rate

It's important for your muscles to recover from session to session. Working one muscle at a time allows that one muscle to rest the next day while working another muscle. However, there are a few flaws in this system. Not only does this mean a full week of workouts, but it also means not having a day for your whole body to rest. When you work out 3-4 days per week, you'll also have 3-4 days off, which will give all of your muscles and your entire central nervous system (CNS)[3] time to rest and recover.

Benefit #3 – More time for the family and other activities

If you're a busy woman, a full body workout is what you need. You'll have more time to spend with the kids, runs errands, etc. because you'll work out your entire body on your workout days and have extra time on your days off.

Benefit #4 – Workout scheduling

A workout schedule can keep you on track, and scheduling a full body workout is a piece of cake. With a full body workout, all you have to do is schedule one workout instead of scheduling a different workout for each day. Say goodbye to scheduling a workout for your abs, arms, etc. The full body workout does it all.

Benefit #5 – Reduce boredom

How many times have you been bored out of your mind while repetitively lifting free weights? If you combine free weights/dumbbells with other exercises, your workout will fly by. You won't have time to look at the clock (admit it, you've done this) and count down the minutes, because your workout will be completed in no time.

Benefit #6 – Great for fat loss

A full body workout is ideal for fat loss, because you work every muscle group at least 3-4 times per week. Combine this with the proper nutrition plan for your body, and you have the perfect formula for greater weight loss.

Benefit #7 – Reduce fatigue

Moving your body, using your muscles, and increasing your heart rate all send your brain a massive message that's quite difficult for your body to ignore: you are awake, and you are alive! This is why working out right before bed prevents people from falling asleep easily. The endorphins running through their bodies are giving them the go-ahead to stay up and put in another ten-hour workday, no sleep needed! Of course, we do need our sleep, which is why starting your day by working out is best.

Benefit #8 – Plateau prevention

Most women get discouraged when they hit a plateau in their weight loss. With *Click it to Rip it*'s full body work-out plan, you won't plateau, because your workouts are constantly changing. You'll enjoy a variety of workouts that will keep you energized and keep you from hitting that plateau.

Benefit #9 – Increase your energy

Once your brain has received that flashing signal that you are awake and alive, your body will get all excited about these great endorphins running through it, telling your brain to keep feeding your body more. The more you work out, the more your endurance will build. The more your endurance builds, the more your body will both want and be able to just keep going!

Benefit #10 – Work out at home

This is a major benefit. You can work out from the comfort of your own home at any time. No more rushing to get to the gym or trying to find a babysitter, if you have kids. You can work out whenever it is most convenient for *you*!

IMPORTANT FITNESS FACTS

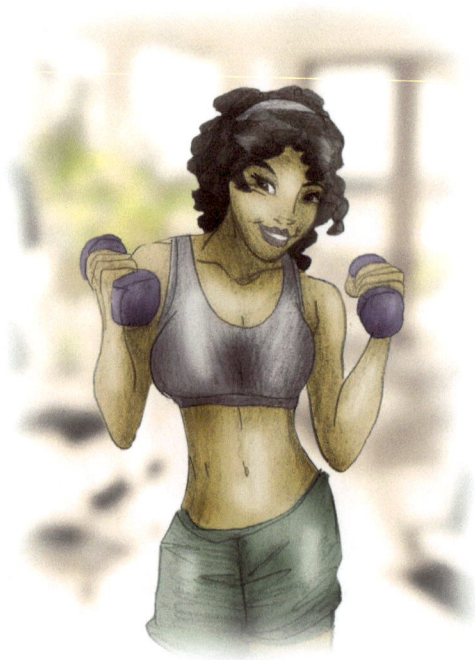

DO YOU WANT TO FEEL less tired? How about improving your mind power? What about eating without feeling guilty? How about spending more time with your family and running around outside with the kids? If you've answered YES to one or more of these questions, working out, losing weight, and getting healthy is the answer.

Being physically fit and active has major benefits. Below are ten fitness facts that will help keep you excited about working out:

Fitness fact #1: Working out boosts your mind power

Serotonin increases in the brain when you work out. This leads to improved mental clarity. How? Serotonin is responsible for moving messages throughout your nervous system.[4] This means that, if you have trouble remembering information, working out can strengthen your brain and your neural connections, which means greater memory capacity.

Fitness fact #2: Working out melts stress in addition to body fat

Have you ever come home from work, wound tighter than a clock? Not only does working out melt body fat, but it also melts stress. There's nothing like working up a sweat to relieve stress and tension. Working out for just 30 minutes can help you forget what got you so worked *up* in the first place!

Fitness fact #3: Working out boosts your mood

You may have heard of the "runner's high" that runners can receive either during or after a run. This is due to endorphins being released into the body. When you work out, these same endorphins, which trigger positive emotions, are released into your body, giving you energy and a more positive outlook on life.

Fitness fact #4: Working out controls and maintains your weight

Think about it. If you continue to eat without moving a muscle, calories are not being burned, and you are sure to gain weight. That is, of course, unless you have a miracle metabolism. Chances are, however, that you don't have this miracle metabolism, which means that you must move your body in order to burn calories. By burning some of the calories that you ingest, you are able to control and maintain your weight.

Fitness fact #5: Working out is fun

Thinking about working out is not necessarily fun. But that's because you haven't started moving your body yet! When you're moving your body, you're releasing those endorphins that we talked about, which means, scientifically, that you're having fun! Plus, you get to listen to your most upbeat music, which will also increase endorphins and fun. And with *Click it to Rip it*, your workouts are always in fun rotation, which means that boredom is not an option!

Fitness fact #6: Working out will improve your sleep

Many people have trouble falling asleep or staying asleep, but working out your entire body 3-4 times per week will actually improve your sleep quality! When you work out in the morning or afternoon (not at night, especially not right before you sleep), your body will feel fulfilled at the end of the day. When your body feels fulfilled, it accepts rest much better and much more easily.

Fitness fact #7: Working out doesn't have to take hours

You don't have to work out for five hours each day like the contestants on weight loss reality shows. Working out anywhere from 20 minutes to one hour, 3-4 times per week, is sufficient. You will lose weight and get healthy in a way that can be sustained for extended periods of time.

Fitness fact #8: Working out can boost your sex life

Working out can boost confidence and eliminate the belly fat that restricts blood flow to sex organs. Women who exercise regularly can enhance their arousal, while men who work out are less likely to have erectile dysfunction.[5]

Fitness fact #9: Working out prevents health conditions and diseases

An increased awareness of the body decreases our chances of unconsciously harming the body. Diet and exercise is an effective way to decrease your chance of cardiovascular disease, depression, arthritis, risk of falling, and so much more.[6] Especially if your family has a history of cancer, stroke, high blood pressure, diabetes, high cholesterol, or heart disease, living a healthy, fit lifestyle is a must.

Fitness fact #10: Working out more means you can eat more

Cutting out pizza, mac and cheese, burgers, alcohol, etc. is a choice that you can always make. However, if you just can't stand to let those foods go, working out will give a little extra wiggle room. If you start and continue to work out 3-4 times per week, you'll be able to enjoy your favorite foods in moderation. Some women like to reserve the weekend for cheat days, where they enjoy their favorite dishes without the guilt. Or, you can modify the recipes of your favorite foods and still eat what you want, only with half the calories.

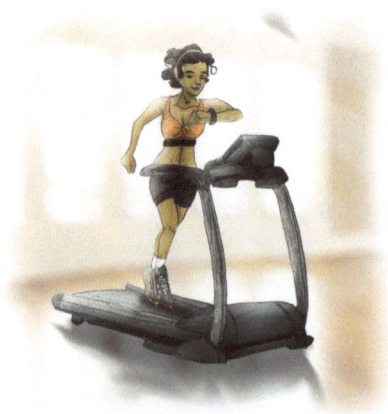

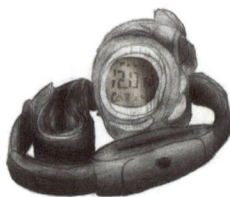

Heart Rate

There are three heart rates (HR's) to consider when training to get fit: resting HR, exercise HR, and maximum HR. In reading the following, you will learn how to calculate each of these HR's, helping you to find your personal target HR in any given zone of fitness activity.

1. Resting HR

This is your HR when you are either in a resting state or are simply not engaging in any physical activity. As you become more fit, the heart and lungs become stronger, allowing the heart to pump more blood with less effort. The volume of blood that pumps through the body per heartbeat is called **stroke volume**. The better the stroke volume, the lower the resting HR.

A normal resting HR can vary from as low as 40 BPM to as high as 100 BPM. The average man rests at 70 BPM, and the average woman rests at 75 BPM. The resting HR should be used as an index to improve your cardiovascular fitness level, with a focus on decreasing it. The best time to measure your resting HR is when you first arise from sleep in the morning. The palpation (beats) of the radial pulse can be accurately measured on the underside of your wrist at the base of your thumb.

1a. How to calculate your resting HR

☐ Place the tips of your index and middle fingers over the radial artery and apply a light pressure. *Do not use your thumb*, because it has a pulse of it's own.

☐ Use a clock, watch, or timer and count your heartbeats for 60 seconds. Always count the first beat as 0.

☐ You will receive the most accurate BPM by counting the beats of your pulse for a full 60 seconds. However, you may also count for 30 seconds and multiply by 2, count for 15 seconds and multiply by 4, count for 10 seconds and multiply by 6, or count for 6 seconds and multiply by 10. Whatever you do, be consistent in the way you count your heartbeat.[7]

2. Exercise HR

This is an increasing HR due to the body being in motion through sustained exercise. Your exercise HR is measured during the time of this sustained exercise and can be most accurately measured at the larger carotid artery on the side of the neck. Place the index and middle fingers alongside the base of the earlobe and slide them down to the side of your throat until you find your pulse. This is your carotid artery. Keep in mind, pressure should be *light*, as these arteries contain baroreceptors that respond to increases in pressure by slowing down your HR. The exercise HR should be taken for 10 seconds, always counting the first beat as 0, then multiplying by 6. The goal of the exercise HR is to stay within your target HR range or zone, which is normally between 75% and 85% of your **maximum HR.**

3. Maximum HR

This is the rate in which your heart beats at 100% max. during a sustained aerobic activity. You do *not* want to work at your maximum HR unless a professional has you on a specifically designed program that your personal fitness level can sustain. Maximum HR will cause you to cross over into an anaerobic threshold. Your maximum HR number will vary depending on your age and fitness level. The best way to find out your maximum HR is to have a treadmill stress test, usually given by your doctor. A doctor will generally recommend a stress test if heart disease or diabetes is in your family history or if you're overweight.

Heart Rate Monitor

Monitoring your heart rate is important when you're trying to lose weight and get healthy. Heart rate monitors are the best, easiest way to measure your intensity so that you can make sure you're reaching your target heart rate zone.[8] The great thing about today's heart rate monitors is that many models are compatible with current workout equipment and can sync up with the equipment's display screen. And when you are not using computerized equipment, heart rate monitors prove great tools for quick, easy, accurate, portable, and perpetual readings of your heart rate. In order to find the right monitor for you, ask your doctor or nutritionist which monitor they would recommend in addition to doing your own research. *Important: if you have a pacemaker, you should not wear a heart monitor.

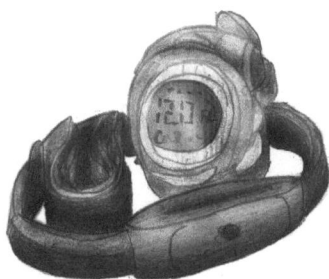

How Does a Heart Rate Monitor Work?

A heart monitor has a chest strap and watch. The chest strap is fastened around the chest with its two sensors placed on each side of the chest. The chest strap senses your heart rate and sends a signal to the watch wirelessly. The watch displays your heart rate in beats per minute. This information can be used to calculate the number of calories you've burned, as well as your maximum heart rate.[9]

Heart rate monitors do come without chest straps. However, information on your pulse is only available when you touch the watch and tends to be less accurate than a monitor with a chest strap.[10]

How to Measure Your Target Heart Rate

The most common way to calculate your Target Heart Rate (THR) is to subtract your age from 226 (for females) or 220 (for males). For example, if you are a 30-year-old female, you will subtract 30 from 226, giving you a Maximum Heart Rate (MHR) of 196. Take this MHR and multiply it by a percentage from one of the five training zones to find your THR.[11]

Training Zones:

Heart Healthy/Warm-up Zone: 50 – 60% of your MHR. This is an easy zone if you're beginning a fitness program. 85 percent of the calories you burn in this zone are fats.[12]

Fitness/Energy Efficient and Recovery Zone: 60 – 70% of your MHR. This is more intense than the warm-up zone and burns more calories. 85 percent of these calories are also fats.[13]

Aerobic Zone: 70 – 80% of your MHR. This zone improves your cardiovascular and respiratory system and increases the strength and capacity of your heart and lungs. You want to be in this zone when you train for an endurance event, because you'll burn more calories. 15 percent of calories from fat are burned.[14]

Anaerobic Zone: 80 – 90% of your MHR. Forget about having a conversation in this zone, because you'll gasp words. You'll improve the following: 1) VO2 maximum or the amount of oxygen you can consume. 2) Cardiorespiratory system. 3) Endurance due to a higher lactate tolerance (you'll be able to better metabolize lactate), which allows you to fight fatigue. 15 percent of calories burned will be from fat.[15]

Red-Line: 90 – 100% of your MHR. This zone burns a lot of calories and is EXTREMELY INTENSE. Most can only stay in this zone for a few minutes. You should only train in this zone if you are in excellent shape. Your doctor should give you the okay before you train in this zone.[16]

Using the example of a 30-year-old woman, whose maximum heart rate is 196 (226 - 30). Let's calculate each zone.

☐ Warm up zone: 50% of 196 (196 x .50) = 98.

☐ Energy efficient zone: 60% of 196 (196 x .60) = 117.6.

☐ Aerobic zone: 70% of 196 (196 x .70) = 137.2.

☐ Anaerobic zone: 80% of 196 (196 x .80)= 156.8.

☐ Red-line: 90% of 196 (196 x .90)= 176.4.

Another method for calculating the maximum heart rate is the Karvonen Formula: The Karvonen Formula uses your resting heart rate (RHR) in the formula (as calculated previously under **Resting HR**). Using the example of a 30-year-old woman, let's calculate a maximum heart rate using the Karvonen Formula:

Lower = 226 – 30 – 75 (Average RHR for females) x .50 (warm-up zone percentage) + 75 (RHR) = 135.5

Higher = 226 – 30 – 75 (RHR) x .70 (endurance training zone percentage) + 75 (RHR) = 159.7

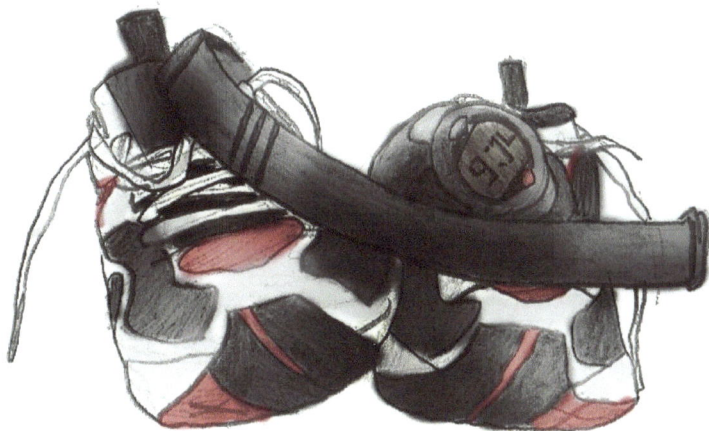

Add Adventure to Your Fitness Journey

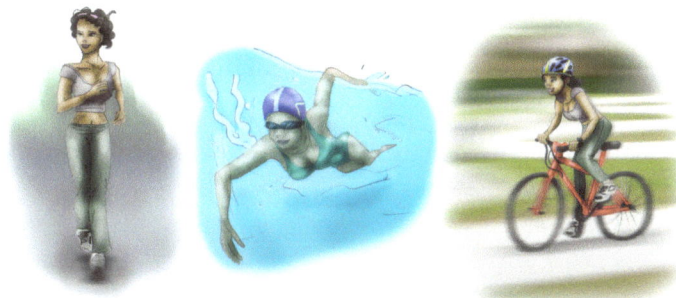

The best part about working from home and doing the *Click it To Rip it* program is that you'll get results from doing YOUR full body workout routine (including cardio). Once you have a set routine, you can always mix in some fun fitness adventures. And remember, fitness never has to be a tedious chore with all of the amazing options out there!

Here's a list of fun workout suggestions:

☐ **If you are someone who enjoys fresh air, beauty, and overcoming challenges**, start going on regular hiking adventures. Bring your friends, and give yourselves a weekend retreat. You deserve it!

☐ **If you enjoy the competitive edge that sports give you**, take up an intramural of your choice. You are sure to meet great people and feel great doing it!

☐ **If you're not one for competition but love to feel the movement of your body**, try out a dance class, yoga, or Pilates. Find a class, or find a DVD. Invite your friends, or find your bliss in solitude.

☐ **If you're one for personal challenges and problem solving**, try out slack lining, bouldering, and rock climbing.

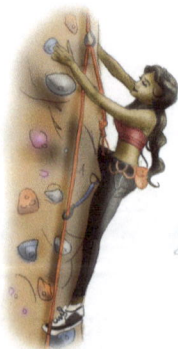

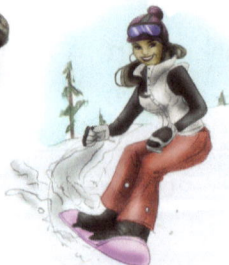

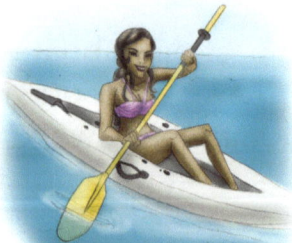

☐ **Add fun, outdoor cardio to your fitness routine, such as running, jogging, swimming, biking, and rollerblading**…and once you've built up your endurance, try one of these:

> ☐ Sign up for a 5k, 10k, half marathon, or a relay race.
>
> ☐ Sign up for a triathlon, or team up with friends and do a triathlon relay (one swim, one bike, and one run).
>
> ☐ Sign up for a bike-a-thon.
>
> ☐ Attend a fitness competition event in your area for some motivation. If it excites you, enter a fitness competition!

The fun doesn't even end here! As the seasons change, options expand infinitely:

☐ **In the winter months**, try out skiing, snowboarding, snowshoeing, ice climbing, or ice-skating!

☐ **In the summer months**, try out some water sports like kayaking, canoeing, whitewater rafting, surfing, kite surfing, swimming, or scuba diving!

Take your journey inward by giving yourself time to relax and meditate daily. Even if you sit silently for only 5 minutes (just 5 minutes out of your entire day!), that can be enough to recharge and center yourself for hours to come.

☐ **If you find yourself with very little extra time on your hands**, you can begin your adventure very easily by incorporating this simple action into everyday life. It's amazing just how invigorated you can feel at the start of your day by simply taking the stairs! Whenever given the option, always take the stairs. If you live or work on the 57th floor of your building, take the stairs a few flights, and then take the elevator. The next day, you might be inspired to climb just a few more!

☐ Take some time to relax and meditate daily.

☐ Schedule an appointment with a dietitian/nutritionist who'll help educate and assist you with your meals and give you some fun food ideas.

☐ Take a nutrition class and healthy cooking class.

☐ Experiment with your meals and shakes; always keep things interesting.

Use Visualization: A Tool for Success

Many successful athletes use visualization to help them win competitions and/or enhance their performance. They exercise their brains by visualizing their goals in their minds (whatever it is they want to achieve), and envisioning the outcome—the positive end result. Napoleon Hill, author of *Think and Grow Rich*, wrote, "What the mind of man can conceive and believe, it can achieve." The power of your mind and thoughts are strong forces, and your thoughts can either motivate or de-motivate you. That on which you focus, you attract. Use the visualization technique to send positive energy to your goals and dreams.

Of course, you can't accomplish your goals through visualization alone. However, visualizing or picturing yourself accomplishing your goal in clear detail increases your chances of making it happen. It improves your focus and concentration, which helps you to remain calm, gain confidence, stay positive, believe, and stay motivated. When you visualize something in which you believe, something realistic, and something that you know you can actually accomplish, it helps to eliminate anxiety, fear, doubt, and negativity.

Below is an example of how I used visualization after being diagnosed with IBS and my food allergies:

For two minutes each morning, five days a week, I visualized myself being pain free. Through this process, I was able to feel better, even just after each of those two minute sessions! After my visualization, I was inspired to eat the foods that would actually keep this pain out of my body for good.

Examples of how you can incorporate visualization into your routine:

Using this same method, you can visualize yourself eating healthy foods and exercising two minutes each morning, five days a week. Visualize yourself enjoying a nutrient rich meal, eating slowly, and feeling your body when it tells you that it's full.

Make it personal!

Whatever your vice is, visualize yourself doing the opposite, and visualize it in detail. For example, if you are a real sucker for sweets, visualize a plate of cookies. Better yet, visualize a plate of *warm* cookies, just out of the oven. They smell amazing, and they're the most tempting cookies you've ever come across. There is even a sign in front of the cookies, written by a loved one, that reads, "Please take one!" Now, visualize yourself walking past this plate of cookies. Visualize yourself having absolutely no desire to put this sugar into your body. Each time you pass the plate of cookies, your desire will continue to decrease.

Let's say your vice is throwing in the towel early when working out. Visualize yourself with a third of your body yet to be worked out, or visualize yourself half-way through your run—whatever the point is in your workout that you feel you're ready to give up for the day. Visualize yourself in detail. You know exactly how you feel when you're about to convince yourself that you can just stop for the day—that you'll just catch up tomorrow...or something. Now, visualize yourself getting a second wind—getting a surge of confidence and motivation. Visualize yourself working out every part of your body until you feel your workout has been thoroughly completed. Lastly, visualize yourself smiling to yourself at your accomplishment. Each time you visualize this scenario, you'll be closer and closer to the point that "throwing in the towel" just doesn't suit you any more.

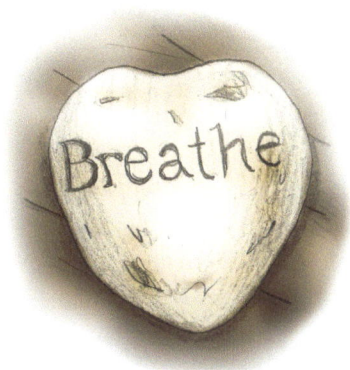

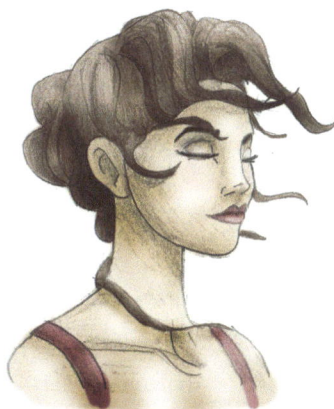

Breathe In and Out Through Your Nose

Oxygen is a major fuel source, and breathing through the nose allows you to take more oxygen into the body, and in a more controlled manner. Practice breathing by inhaling and exhaling through your nose, or better yet, make this a habit. Inhaling and exhaling through your nose is extremely healthy and has many benefits. Here are just a few:

☐ Relieves stress and anxiety.

☐ Reduces hyperventilation and hypertension.

☐ Limits air intake, forcing you to slow down and center yourself.

☐ Stimulates your digestive system.

☐ Increases oxygen in your blood with each inhalation. This benefits your lungs, brain, and body as a whole.

☐ Reduces seasonal allergies, as you're filtering air that is inhaled to the lungs, keeping allergenic particles out of your body.

☐ Controls asthma symptoms.

☐ Helps you to sleep better.

Fun Fact: Athletes inhale and exhale through their noses to help their performance.

Motivation and Inspiration From My Registered Dietician, Colleen Grossner

"Once a great man, my grad school adviser, Marco Cabrera, may he rest in peace, gave me a compliment that I've always remembered. He said, 'you're (me) not afraid to fail.' Didn't seem like much of a compliment at the moment, but in the years since, I've found that this is an attribute of many successful people in history. If you go for what's beyond what you KNOW you can achieve, you'll reach for really amazing goals and awesome possibilities, with some failures, and other seemingly impossible accomplishments, and always truly exciting experiences!" Colleen Grossner, MS, RD, LD

On her blog, *Fresh You*[17] Colleen shares fun food ideas and more amazing information to help you on your way to a healthy and fit lifestyle.

5 Things to Have While Training

These are the five things I always carry with me when training:

☐ **Fitness journal.** In my fitness journal, I write down my training and diet. This practice keeps me in check with my goals, helps keep me accountable, and allows me to track my progress.

☐ **Water bottle.** It's extremely important to *stay hydrated* when you work out, which is why I always carry a water bottle with me. I love water!

☐ **Fully charged tablet/mp3 player/mobile device.** Electronics can be so wonderful! With my tablet, I'm able to read or listen to motivating music, which enables me to beat the treadmill boredom!

☐ **Workout gloves.** Workout gloves help by keeping my hands blister-free and by giving me a good grip while holding my dumbbells or free weights.

☐ **Positive attitude!** Mind over matter, ladies! I always pump myself up with a positive attitude, both before entering, and all throughout my workout. Working out is fun, and living this fit lifestyle feels flippin' fabulous!

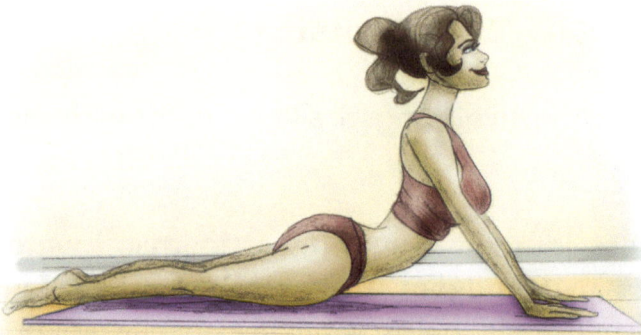

Improve Your Overall Well-Being by Doing the Following

Let's face it; we only have so much time on this earth to do what we want to do and be who we want to be. You are responsible for your overall well-being, and you are the only person who can make profound and drastic changes within yourself. It's time to start taking action! It's time to take back your life and start living again! Below are some tips to help you improve your quality of life RIGHT NOW:

- ☐ **Meditation.** Just as the muscles in our bodies need time to rest, our brains also need time to rest. We may have to remind ourselves to take time to work out our biceps and abs, but our brains are the ones with the real body builder's mentality—they are working out 24/7! When we give our minds a rest, we are able to better organize our thoughts, think more clearly, and use these body builder brains far more effectively. The mind is a powerful tool, and when we are able to observe our thoughts without attachment or judgment, we are capable of great feats. Meditation is a path that also builds on itself, giving us increasingly more unique metaphysical experiences that can't happen unless we quiet the mind or practice mindfulness.

- ☐ **Sleep.** Giving our brains time to rest is very important—did I mention that already? Well, just in case the message didn't stick, I'll say it again: giving ourselves time to rest is *very important!* It may seem counterproductive to take time out of our never-ending schedules to do absolutely nothing, but it's often those confusing and fascinating paradoxes in life that end up giving us the most effective results. Giving your brain and body the amount of sleep they require will help you stay more alert and use your time more effectively when you are awake. Sleeping also aids in metabolism and weight loss, keeps you looking and feeling younger, and helps keep you in good health.

Make sleep one of your top priorities so that your waking life can be spent *fully* awake.

☐ **Yoga.** Practicing yoga will improve flexibility, circulation, strength, posture, mindfulness, and awareness of the body, among many other benefits. Yoga is a great way to start your workout, end your workout, to do in tandem with meditation, and/or to do on the days you're not working out. Yoga is your time to listen to your body and feel what it needs. Especially when using your muscles in aerobic activity, your muscles need to be stretched and relaxed. Doing yoga will elongate your muscles, teach you how to breathe into your muscles, and increase balance. When you are able to feel the needs of your body, you are better able to serve your body and serve yourself.

Set SMART Goals

Goals are powerful! They are motivating and, once completed, give you a sense of achievement. **Goals are essential in helping you be successful, especially when they are SMART: Specific, Measurable, Achievable, Realistic, and Timely.** SMART goals keep you focused on what you want to accomplish:

☐ **Specific.** When you make specific goals, you leave far less wiggle room. You don't need to be extremely rigid with yourself, but giving yourself some guidelines can help greatly in your success. Simply saying,

"I want to start working out," could mean a number of things. Accomplishing that goal could mean doing something as little as ten push-ups once a week. If doing ten push-ups once a week is what you really define as working out, then that's great, and your specific goal should be to do ten push-ups once a week. However, if that isn't really your idea of a fulfilling workout goal, then you need to give yourself something more specific and more personally fulfilling to work towards: "I want to do a full body workout for one hour a day, four days a week."

☐ **Measurable.** Give yourself numbers and figures with which to work. Once again, *I want to start working out* is vague and doesn't provide you with any concrete data like "one hour" or "four days a week." Your figures could be "30 minutes to an hour" or "three to four days a week," giving yourself some room for outlying factors. However, you're giving yourself something measurable, to which you can turn for guidance and inspiration.

☐ **Achievable.** Let's say you want to look like a celebrity who you admire. This may not be what you what you want to hear, but if she has an hourglass shaped body and you have an apple shaped body, you can get down to a weight that is *less* that that of this celebrity and never have a single similar feature. But that's what makes you unique and wonderful! Embrace your body and use your *own* body as inspiration for achievable goals.

☐ **Realistic.** Telling yourself that you're going to work out for 14 hours a day, seven days a week is 1) likely something that that has ever crossed the mind of maybe three people on the planet and 2) not realistic...for many reasons that you can ponder on your own. Cramming your workouts, much like cramming for a test, doesn't actually work. Be realistic about your goals.

☐ **Timely.** On the other hand, let's say you want to lose 50 pounds and are only working out one day a week. If you *really* want to lose 50 pounds, you're not going to want a workout plan that will make you take years to achieve your goal. Give yourself a reasonable time line. Let your timeline be flexible, because not everyone's metabolism or weight starts out the same, meaning that not everyone is going to lose weight at the same rate. Once you get to know your body a little better through working out, you can give yourself a realistic timeline for your weight loss and workout goals.

Chuck-Out the Plastics

Help heal the planet, and help heal yourself by getting rid of those plastics! Recycle your plastic bottles and containers, and replace them with glass ones. Plastic utensils, containers, etc. release chemicals into your body, which can be harmful to your health. Instead of using a plastic cutting board, use a wood cutting board instead. Aim to eliminate the use of plastic in materials that can easily be ingested into the body.

Tips for Living a Happy Life

Outlying circumstances are merely obstacles when it comes to happiness. Believe it or not, living a happy life is a decision, and that decision is *yours*. **Here are some tips for living a happier life:**

☐ **Make yourself a priority.** While taking care of, loving, and giving to others is wonderful, you will care, love, and give far more genuinely when you love yourself. Just as a relationship with someone else takes time and work, so does a relationship with yourself—and you are 100 percent guaranteed to live with yourself your *entire life*, which means that this is your longest and most important relationship to maintain. Take time to yourself every day to do what you love and to do what makes you feel fulfilled—sometimes, taking time to do absolutely nothing and to feel comfort in silence is all the fulfillment you'll need.

☐ **Be grateful.** Gratitude is bliss, and no matter what you have or don't have, there is always something for which to be grateful. Try out these exercises to improve gratitude:

Every morning when you wake up, or every night before you go to bed, write down five things that make you grateful. Read over the list as many times as is necessary to feel profoundly grateful for those five things. Why did you choose those five today, out of everything else in your life, for which to be grateful?

Go through all of your clothing, your jewelry—all your *stuff*—and find at least five things to give away. As you go through every item you choose to keep, practice gratitude for this item.

Do a meditation, choosing at least five people on whom to concentrate—you can challenge yourself by including people with whom you have difficulty understanding or seeing eye-to-eye. Begin with yourself. List at least five reasons that you're grateful to yourself. Send good wishes and love to yourself. Then, go through your list of five or more people and do the same, sending love and gratitude to each person.

☐ **Be positive.** From now on, build awareness every time you think negatively or speak negatively (especially about yourself). When we have a positive self-image, we tend to think positively about those around us. When we think, speak, and act positively, those around us tend to be more positive as well. You can incorporate positivity and positive thoughts into the exercises listed above.

☐ **Lead by example.** Inspire your loved ones and all those around you. Do what you admire, and feel fulfillment in doing it. Being that you are here, chances are pretty good that you admire those who lead healthy, fit lifestyles, and it just so happens that leading this kind of lifestyle can be one of the most inspiring things you can do—both for yourself and others.

☐ **Surround yourself** with good, positive people who treat others well. Be accepting of others, and appreciate people for who they are, even if (especially if) they're not the people with whom you chose to surround yourself. By being open, you are opening others to your way of being.

☐ **Forgive yourself** for anything for which you've been hard on yourself—especially matters of the past. Learn from your mistakes and live for the present, knowing that you are always doing your best, trying your hardest, and putting your best foot forward.

☐ **Volunteer.** Do something for someone else, including friends, acquaintances, and strangers. Volunteer your time, compassion, words of encouragement, and compliments.

☐ **Laugh often!** Allow happiness to permeate and resonate through laughter—one of life's greatest over the counter remedies (or something like that). Life can be funny, silly, ironic—you name it. Don't be afraid to let go and allow laughter to be your medicine.

THE WOMAN'S BODY

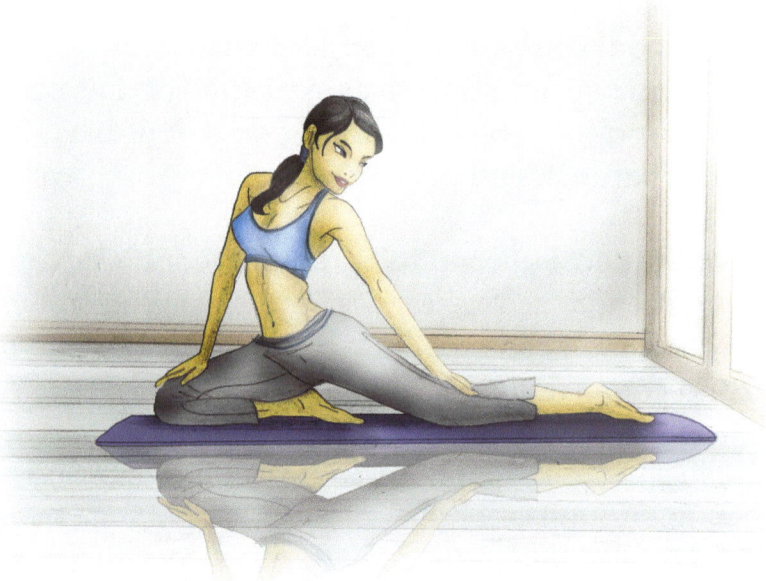

THE WOMAN'S BODY IS NARROWER at the waist than it is at the bust and hips, and the ratio of the bust, hips, and waist is used to define a woman's shape. This is just one fascinating and fun fact about a woman's body. Here are some others:

☐ Women have a good sense of smell. They can generally detect smells better than men.[18]

☐ Due to hormones, women generally have a great deal less body hair than men.[19]

☐ Women's arms tend to be shorter, less muscular, and more slender than a man's arms.[20]

☐ The shoulders of women tend to be more slender than a man's shoulders.[21]

☐ Women tend to lose collagen in their skin faster than men due to hormonal changes. The good news is that women look younger in photos![22]

☐ Women have guts! Men and women have the same digestive organs (stomach, liver, gallbladder, colon), but women have a longer sigmoid (lower portion of the colon).Plus, women's lower bodies are filled with reproductive organs.[23]

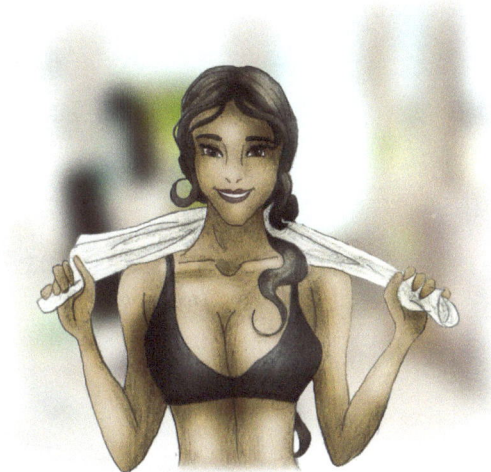

How to Train the Woman's Body

"Movement is medicine for changing a person's physical, emotional, and mental state." – Carol Welch.

In this section, I'm going to teach you *how* to move in a way that is medicinal. You may be thinking, "What type of exercises should I do to train my body?" Any exercise you do is better than doing nothing at all. But I suggest an all-over body workout that combines strength training and cardio. Not only will you lose weight, but you'll also build lean muscle and endurance.

Strength training exercises include:

☐ Bending

☐ Twisting

☐ Pushing and pulling

☐ Stretching

☐ Lunging

Cardio training (also known as conditioning training) exercises include:

☐ Running

☐ Treadmill sprints

☐ BOSU® ball

☐ Weight lifting (10 lbs. or more)

☐ Elliptical

☐ Kickboxing

☐ Walking

☐ Jumping rope

You may be thinking, "If I lift heavy weights will I get big and bulky?"No, you will not get big and bulky. Testosterone is what aids in building bulk. Being that you are a woman, your testosterone level is merely a fraction of a man's.[24] What's that you say? You didn't know you had testosterone? You bet your booty you do!

A man's testosterone level is 200-1200 ng/dl, and a woman's normal level is 15-70 ng/dl.[25] So you see, it would be very difficult for you to bulk up unless you were to take exogenous testosterone injections and/or other anabolic steroids. Through the full body workout program, you should be building and gaining lean muscle, giving you a sculpted look. You can achieve this by lifting weights and doing at least three sets of 15-20 reps. Remember, lifting weights will be done in conjunction with other exercises.

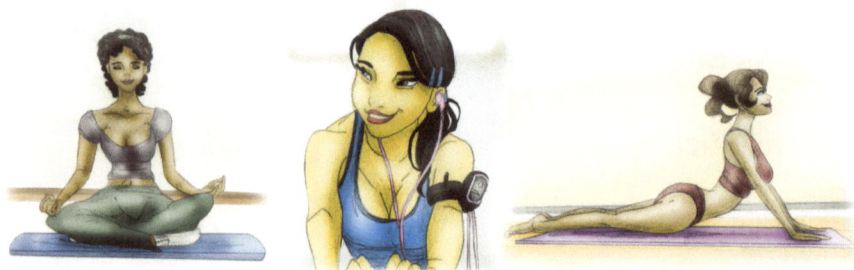

The Most Common Mistakes That Gym Goers Make

Most gym goers, including myself, are clueless when it comes to starting to work out at the gym. See if this sounds like you:

You've worked out day after day and week after week, in addition to cutting calories and drinking more water, but you still haven't lost any weight. It's frustrating and you probably want to give up.

Most women who work out at the gym are making these four common mistakes:[26]

☐ Working out using cardio equipment that isn't as effective as other workout equipment or exercises.

☐ Focusing solely on cardio and either foregoing or doing too little strength and resistance training

☐ Lifting weights too quickly (something that happens when weights are intimidating, too heavy, or too light for the lifter)

☐ Performing too many sets/reps per exercise

While there is nothing wrong with using the elliptical machine or treadmill, you'll want to incorporate resistance and weight training as well. When choosing your weights, find weights that neither prove difficult to lift off of the floor initially, nor are so easy to lift that they surprisingly fly off the shelf in your grasp. In your exercises, try 2-3 sets of 12 reps each instead of 4 or 5 sets. All of these tips will help greatly at the gym, but will also help greatly with your new home workout regiment.

The reason that many women are misinformed when going to the gym is simple: the primary job of the gym's sales team is not to be your personal trainer. The primary job of the gym's sales team is to get members to sign up—that's it. They don't care if you never go back to the gym again, because their focus is on making their monthly, quarterly, and yearly sales. And, if 30 percent of members actually showed up at the gym, this would be a HUGE problem. Members would have to wait in long lines to use the equipment, and nobody would leave very happy. It would be total chaos![27]

Women also become misinformed when the majority of their information comes in short snippets from fitness magazines that teach you how to "melt away the fat without sweating" and to "tone your trouble zone." Many women are missing the full picture by treating fitness regiments as fads. But you know better, which is why you're here! Fitness is not a fad that changes from week to week. Fitness is a long-term lifestyle change that should be unique to each practitioner.

The Personal Trainer's Perspective

Fitness coach, writer, and mom, Neghar Fonooni, has been helping women transform their lives and become the best possible versions of themselves for over 12 years. She says, "I have witnessed, in awe and admiration, the tremendous work ethic and perseverance of RKC (Russian Kettlebell Challenge) women. These are women who don't believe that serious strength and conditioning is limited to men. These are women who believe in their ability to use their bodies in exceptional ways, who exceed limits imposed by the fitness mainstream and harbor a mental toughness that propels and motivates them."[28]

As your personal fitness coach, it is my job to help you see that you are powerful in your mind and body. Being an athlete, or even just being someone who works out, isn't just about physical feats or aesthetic goals. It's about creating a strong self-image, gaining self-confidence, developing an empowering attitude, and getting a sense of satisfaction from completing a workout. When you do the work to see what you and your body are capable of, you have no one but yourself to thank.

While I am here to help motivate and inform you, it is also your job to motivate yourself and to hold yourself accountable. I'm not going to know whether or not you're working out 3-4 times a week, which means that your personal transformation is entirely in your power. You are able to feel the satisfaction of knowing that it's YOU who is pushing yourself to make this change. It's YOU who's making the decision to eat healthy and to test your limits.

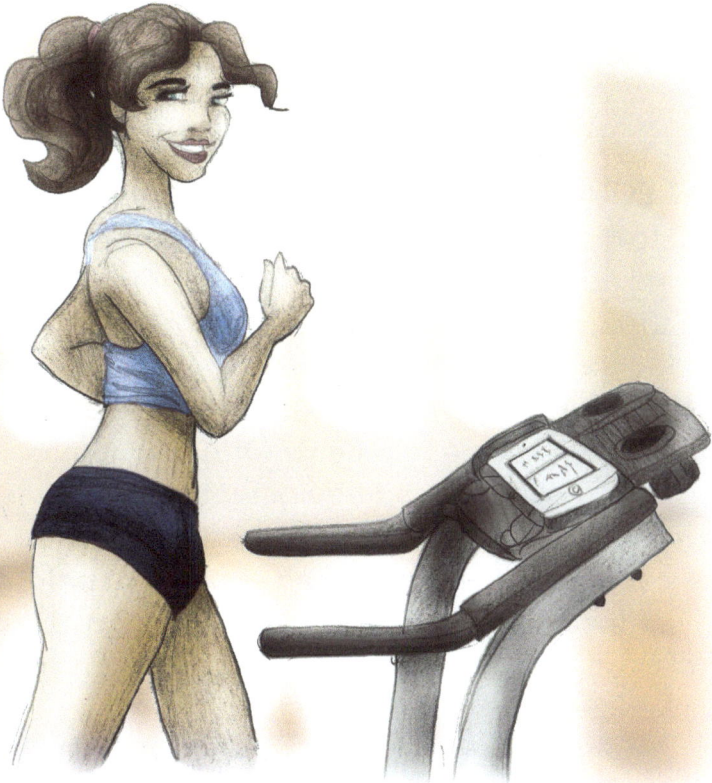

WORKOUT EQUIPMENT

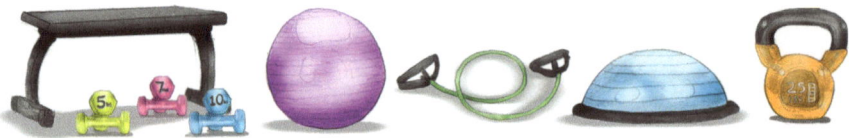

WHAT EQUIPMENT DO YOU NEED to work out? With the *Click it to Rip it* app, you can have a completely fulfilling workout using no equipment at all! However, it may be in your interest to invest in some other equipment I recommend here.

Believe it or not, you don't have to spend thousands of dollars on workout equipment. Often times the best option is to buy slightly used equipment from your neighbor's garage sale or online. It may or may not surprise you that some people will *hardly use their equipment* before putting it online for half the price! And when *you* put this equipment to use, it will end up being far more worth it than the annual price of a gym membership.

One of the best parts about working out at home with your own equipment is that you are avoiding the massive amount of germs you'd otherwise encounter at the gym.

At the gym, everyone sweats, and everyone sweats on the equipment they use. Unfortunately, not everyone wipes down that equipment. Gross! And even if members do wipe down workout equipment once or twice, there's still a potential for germs to be hanging around that equipment.[29] Sanitizing your own equipment is good practice, but even if you don't, at least you know that it has your sweat on it and not the sweat of 30 different people!

Workout Equipment

☐ **Dumbbells / Free Weights**

According to the Physical Activity Guidelines for Americans, "You need both aerobic and muscle-strengthening exercise every week. The recommendation is to include muscle strengthening at least two days a week.[30]"

Resistance or strength training is when you use your muscles against some type of resistance. Free weights and other strength training equipment are the most common ways to incorporate resistance or strength training into your full body workout. This is an important part of weight loss for women. You'll **improve muscle strength** and **endurance** along with **heart health**, **bone strength**, **balance**, and **coordination**. Remember, as you age, you lose muscle. Building or maintaining this muscle is important, and incorporating resistance/strength training into your workouts is one of the best ways to do this.[31]

Like women, free weights come in all shapes in sizes. You can use a pair of dumbbells/free weights together or individually. You can choose to get a large set of weights or to get just one or two pairs. Some weights have a protective rubber coating while others do not. Some weights are ergonomically designed for your comfort, while others are not. Some come in fun, vibrant colors, while others, you guessed it, do not. There are many options from which to choose, so choose whatever works best for you. There's no need, however, to get too caught up in all the fancy shapes and styles. The most important part is picking a set of weights that's comfortable for you in both size and, well, weight!

The best way to determine the most useful weight of your bumbbells/free weights is by setting them onto the ground in front of you. If you can't lift the weights off of the floor again, these are definitely not for you. If you can lift the weights but struggle to do so, these weights are also not for you. If you go to pick up the weights and find that they fly up with you as you lift your body back up, then these weights are not for you either. Find a pair of weights that you can lift comfortably off of the ground, and these will be the best weights with which to do the majority of your reps and sets. Just keep in mind that, as you get stronger (and you will get stronger), you'll want to increase your weights!

☐ **Swiss Ball / Stability Ball**

Swiss balls are known by a variety of names, such as stability ball, exercise ball, gym ball, Pilates ball, sports ball, fitness ball, therapy ball, yoga ball, balance ball, body ball, or birth ball. Whew! Ok, now part of your training is to say that all in one breath… just kidding. Essentially, a Swiss ball is a heavy-duty inflatable ball, usually with a diameter of 45 to 75 cm (18 to 30 inches).[32] Swiss balls are extremely durable, giving you a long exercise life, in addition to being one of the least expensive pieces of workout equipment.

☐ **Kettlebell**

The kettlebell is a low-tech piece of equipment that basically looks like a cannonball with a handle. The kettlebell originated in Russia in the 1700s with the same purpose as its use today: weight training and competitions.[33] Like free weights and dumbbells, kettlebells come in a variety of colors and weights from which to choose.

☐ **Weight Bands**

Weight bands, resistance bands, or tubing are great for strength training, just like free weights, dumbbells, and kettlebells. The weight bands are basically giant rubber bands that are used to create resistance and to strengthen and work out certain muscle groups.[34]

They come in a variety of colors, sizes, and resistance levels and are easy to pack in your suitcase when you travel.

Use weight bands or resistance bands to target specific areas, such as your hamstrings. Place a weight band around your ankle and perform butt and leg kicks as you hold on to a safe and secure surface.[35] Always remember to stretch your legs and body after you've worked out.

☐ **Flat Bench**

A flat bench is a very basic structure with a steel frame and a slightly cushioned foam board, usually covered in vinyl. The flat bench is used in certain workouts that require sitting or laying on an elevated surface.[36] It can be used in conjunction with free weights and is great for adding variation to your workouts. For example, you can do abdominal crunches, as well as chest, back, and leg exercises in fuller motion than you could just laying on the floor.

☐ **BOSU® Ball**

The BOSU® ball is essentially an exercise ball that's been cut in half and placed on a platform, making it form the shape of a dome. The BOSU® ball is extremely versatile and gives you many exercise options and benefits. For example, if you flip it over and use the platform side, you can do push-ups or planks with the added challenge of balance. If you use the ball side, you can do core moves, cardio, and lower-body moves such as leaps, lunges, stepping, crunches, etc.[37] You can even improve your flexibility and balance simultaneously by standing on the dome side while stretching. Now that's a challenge!

The BOSU® ball will primarily help with balance, general awareness, kinesthetic awareness, and proprioception or the way in which your body responds to an external force. The BOSU® ball can be used to enhance your step aerobics, yoga, and a number of other exercise regiments.

☐ **Medicine Ball**

A medicine ball is a weighted ball that's used in exercises that strengthen the arms, core, and back. It too can be used for a wide variety of exercises and is especially good for partner exercises. For example, you can throw the ball to a partner while doing crunches, giving you an added challenge of weight, awareness, and concentration. The medicine ball is also great for solo abdominal crunches and will provide you with the same benefits.[38]

☐ **Workout / Exercise Mats**

There is a wide variety of workout mats, and it's important to select the right one for you. You want the right amount of support for any given workout. **Here are the top styles of work out mats:**

☐ **Pilates and Yoga**

Pilates and yoga mats are similar. However, a Pilates mat is longer and thicker (at least half an inch thick) and isn't sticky like a yoga mat. It is generally made from TPE (Thermal Plastic Elastomer) and wipes clean easily after use. Yoga mats can be made from closed cell PVC, cotton, mesh, and rubber, and they cling to a floor in order to keep from slipping out from under you. They can be cleaned easily with soap and water.[39]

☐ **Fitness**

Fitness mats are thick and large, generally about five feet long and at least a half an inch thick. Fitness mats are used for abdominal crunches and stretching exercises, because they provide your body with a cushion and absorb some impact shock. A fitness mat usually has an easy to clean vinyl cover.[40]

☐ **Foam**

Foam mats are two by two feet, interlocking mats that are generally about five inches thick. They are used for martial arts classes and high intensity exercise classes.[41]

☐ Floor Protectors

Floor protectors are used to protect a floor from exercise equipment, such as stationery bike, rowing machine, treadmill, elliptical, home gym, weights, etc. Floor protectors can be over eight feet long and three feet wide and should be non-slip.[42] They can be one piece or interlocking and are usually made of vinyl or carpet.

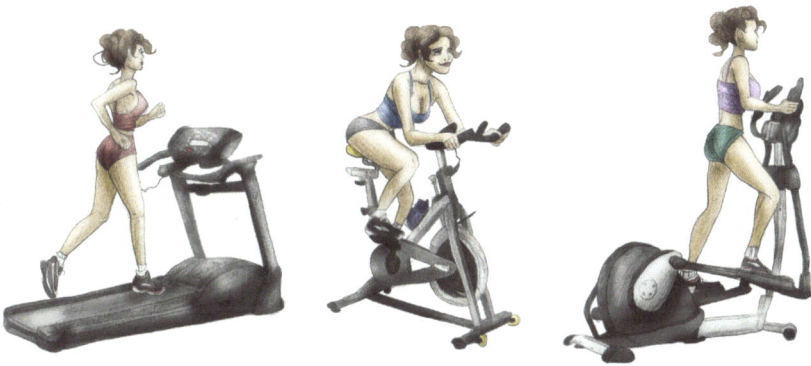

Cardio Equipment

Cardio equipment comes in a wide variety of styles, from high-tech to low-tech. **Below are the top pieces of cardio equipment:**

☐ Treadmill

Treadmills have been around for quite some time, and are just as effective now as when they first emerged.[43] The treadmill features a conveyor-style belt that allows you to run, jog, sprint, or walk. You can find a treadmill new or used, though I always recommend the used equipment. You don't need anything fancy like the ones at the gym—just something that will allow you to run in the comfort of your own home. However, you can definitely find some pretty snazzy, gently used equipment out there!

☐ **Elliptical**

The elliptical trainer or cross trainer entered the fitness market in 1990. Ellipticals feature two foot pedals and two handles (which work out the upper body in addition to the lower) that allow you to move your body in an 'elliptical' motion. The intensity can be low or high by adjusting the incline and resistance, and the elliptical can be used at the speed of your choice. The elliptical simulates the sensation of stair climbing, running, and walking without putting added pressure on joints, which reduces injuries. This makes the elliptical a non-impact cardio workout machine.

☐ **Bike (stationery and regular)**

Riding a bike is a great cardio workout and can be done in the excitement of the outdoors or in the comfort of your own home. Not only is riding a bike (regular or stationary), easy to do, but it's also a fun exercise. Outdoor bikes come in a variety of styles and are intended for many different terrains and biking styles. Here are some examples:

☐ Standard bike

☐ Mountain bike

☐ Racing bike

☐ Touring bike

☐ Triathlon bike

☐ BMX bike

There are also a few different types of stationary bikes. Some are high-tech, while others are low-tech. There are upright bikes and recumbent style bikes (the type you pedal from a reclined position).[44] There are also used bikes and new bikes. Stationary bikes tend to be easy on the joints and prove a good piece of workout equipment for beginners. The other wonderful thing about stationary bikes is that you don't have to prepare for or be stopped by the weather. In making your final decision, ask around and do your research. Find what works best for you.

☐ Stair Climbers/Steppers

An exercise stepper can be a fun way to work out, lose weight, and get fit by toning and strengthening muscles. A stepper has two stepping pedals that provide resistance, as you climb continually upward while simultaneously staying in one place. Some steppers are portable, while others can take up a great deal of space.

The stepper may be a low impact piece of workout equipment, but when you combine it with other work-out equipment such as free weights, weight bands, or a stability ball, you can really kick it up a notch and have a great workout.

☐ **Air Walker**

The air walker is a piece of workout equipment that is constructed out of strong steel; it has a steel frame with two handles and two foot pedals. While holding yourself up on the handles, you move the foot pedals back and forth, as if you're walking on air. By incor-porating your upper body in this way, you'll receive a low impact cardio workout that will tone your en-tire body and help you to lose weight. The air walker comes in a variety of designs and isn't specific to one manufacturer.

☐ **Home Gym**

A home gym or multi-gym is a compact piece of workout equipment that allows you to do more than one exercise in one place. For example, you can lift weights, which will work any number of muscles in the arms, while doing core exercises and/or leg exer-cises. The options are nearly infinite.

The idea behind the home gym is that you have an entire gym of equipment rolled into one, convenient piece of equipment that can be used in the comfort of your own home. Home gyms come in a wide variety of complexities and prices. Always do your research, and investigate the used market before deciding that you need something new.

Once again, these different pieces of equipment are just examples of what you can add to your home workout. Don't let this list intimidate you, and please don't feel like you have to go out and buy every piece of workout equipment on the market. You may feel completely fulfilled without any equipment, and that's great! If, however, you'd like to start incorporating more tools into your workout regiment, start slowly by getting the first couple of items on the list or by complementing the equipment you already have. If you already use a Swiss ball and love it, then you'll probably really enjoy using a BOSU® ball. If you love biking but don't want to bike outside during the colder months, continue your biking inside on a stationary bike!

Comfortable Workout Clothes That Fit

If you're not wearing comfortable workout clothes, you won't enjoy working out. In fact, buying a new workout outfit and shoes is a great motivator to help you start your workouts and stick with them. **Here's a list of items that you'll need:**

☐ **Sports Bra**

Breasts are one of the areas that make our shapes so unique, and finding the right support for your unique shape is extremely important. It's just as important to select the right sports bra as it is your regular bra. Like a regular bra, a sports bra should fit across your back without riding up, and your breasts should not droop. A sports bra should hold your breasts in place without causing pain or squishing your breasts. Sports bras with an underwire work well at holding you in place, especially if you have large breasts.

If you have difficulty finding a good sports bra, ask a women's associate at a sporting goods store to help you select the right bra for you. Some large retail stores also sell sports bras and have a brassier con-sultant on hand to help women find the right bra.

☐ **Athletic Socks**

The socks you put on your feet are just as important as the shoes you wear, because they protect your feet when you work out. Going to the gym? Wearing socks protects your feet from fungus and other germs. Cotton fibers will absorb moisture and pro-vide a cooling effect on the feet, holding the mois-ture against the skin, whereas synthetic fibers help to wick away moisture from the feet, keeping them dry. For the everyday workout, I would recommend synthetic fibers for this reason. If you're going hiking or are working out in colder weather, wool socks will absorb moisture beautifully while keeping your feet warm.[45]

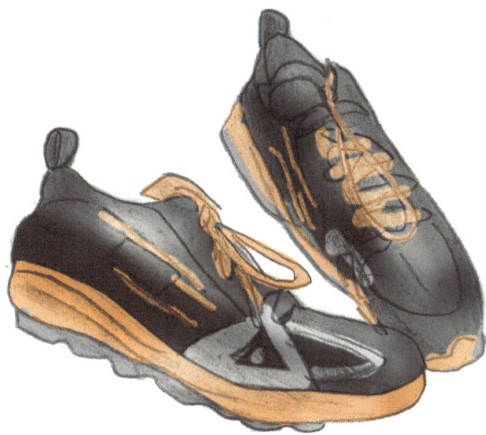

☐ **Comfortable Athletic/Workout Shoes**

Shoes are probably the most important article that we put onto our bodies, because they're where we place all of our weight whenever we're standing, walking, running, etc. Wearing improper shoes can result in knee problems, back problems, shin splints, etc., so take your time in selecting the right pair of shoes. Walk around the store, making sure to walk on a non-carpeted area to test the true comfort of the shoes (carpeting provides extra cushioning, which often tricks us into thinking that shoes are far more comfortable than they really are).

There are many different brands on the market, as well as many different types of shoes. Cross trainers are best for all workout activities, but if you're doing a specific sport regularly, buy shoes that are specifically made for that sport (i.e. running shoes for running).

Your shoes should be comfortable. They should have a toe box that's wide enough and high enough for your toes to move around comfortably. There should be enough cushioning and support in the toe boxes, in the arches, and in the heels. Shoes should be fitted (but not tight) at the ankle, holding the ankle in place and holding your shoe onto your foot.

If you can't find something that serves your feet and your body well, ask your doctor about orthotics. Custom orthotics can fix a vast number of problems that you may not have even known stemmed from wearing improper shoes.

☐ **Workout Clothing**

Workout clothing comes in a variety of colors and fabrics, such as cotton, wool, polyester, and spandex. Cotton is a great fiber when it is loosely fitted, because it absorbs moisture and is extremely breathable. When tightly fitted, cotton can be uncomfortable, because it can hold the moisture it absorbs against the skin. This can cause chafing and, in some cases, yeast infections.[46] Synthetic fibers (i.e. polyester and spandex) are less breathable but are able to wick moisture away from the body, keeping you dry when you work out. The other wonderful thing about synthetic fibers is that they can both be made from recycled plastic and are recyclable themselves. The tighter woven a fabric is and the closer the fabric is to the body, the warmer you will be. Dressing in tightly woven layers, or dressing in thin wool layers will also keep you extremely warm and dry. Wool, like cotton, is also much more breathable than synthetic fibers. Unlike cotton, however, wool dries very quickly and does not hold moisture against the body.

When working out, embrace sweat! Sweating is great for getting out toxins and for naturally cooling down the body. However, if you know that you sweat an uncomfortable amount when working out, find a looser fitting garment with a more breathable fabric, like mesh, which generally comes in the synthetic fibers that will wick moisture away from your body.[47]

Select workout clothing, sports bras, shoes, and socks that are right for YOUR BODY. If you're not comfortable in your clothes, you won't be motivated to workout. Workout clothes don't need to show off every piece of your body, but workout clothes tend to make the movement of your body easier when they are fitted closer to your skin. When clothes are too loosely fitted, they tend to fly up and get in the way, showing off more than you had intended anyways. Close fitting workout clothes can also decrease muscle tension, because your entire body is kept more snuggly in place. Remember, your appearance can be the last thing on your mind when doing your workouts from home! And in a couple of weeks, who knows! Maybe you'll [gasp] WANT to take a run around the neighborhood with your hot self!

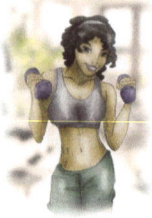

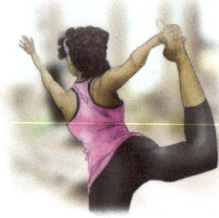

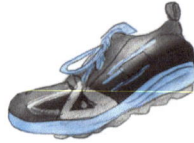

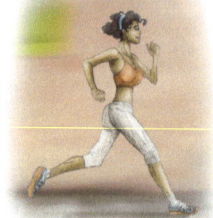

HOW TO STAY MOTIVATED

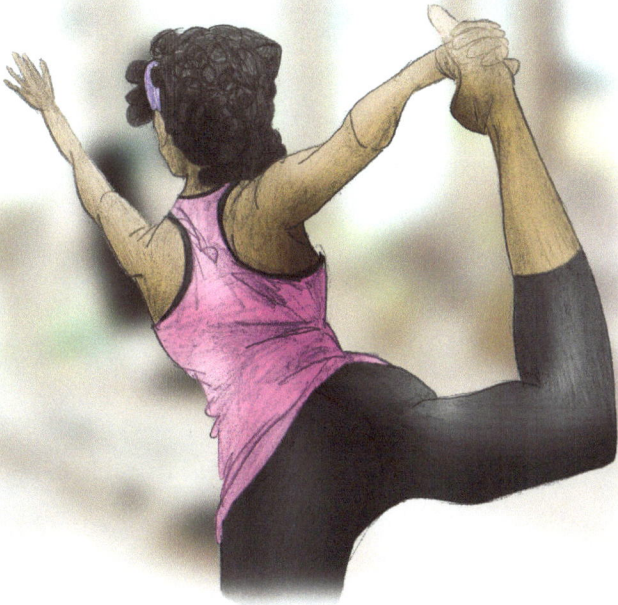

LOSING WEIGHT AND KEEPING IT OFF takes discipline and motivation. When I first decided to start exercising and changing my lifestyle, I had to develop little tricks to keep myself motivated and to keep myself moving forward. In this section, I'm going to share with you how I stayed motivated when I began my fitness journey, and how I continue to stay motivated to this day.

Fitness Journal

In the beginning of my fitness journey, I sat down and mapped out my plan. I wrote down my goals, what I wanted to accomplish, and why. This helped give me clarity about my situation and where I wanted to be.

A few of the things I listed in my journal:

☐ I want to be comfortable and confident in my body. I want to embrace my height [4′ 11″], shape, and size. I want to really appreciate what I have.

☐ I'm tired of spending money on clothing to make me feel good about myself. I don't want to use shopping as a form of therapy any more.

☐ I want to have more energy and feel lighter, not sluggish.

☐ I want to do this for my family and the people around me. I want to be a positive influence by making better choices for my health and lifestyle.

After getting in shape, I felt confident enough in my body that I didn't need to go shopping as a form of therapy. I just felt good about myself all the time, no matter what my outfit. I have more energy and make better choices regarding my health and lifestyle, and by making these choices, I help to motivate and influence those around me.

Your reasons for getting into shape and starting your own fitness journey may differ, but it's important to get a clear understanding of where you are and where you want to be. Write down your goals in a special fitness journal or notebook. Laying everything out on the table for yourself is empowering and motivating.

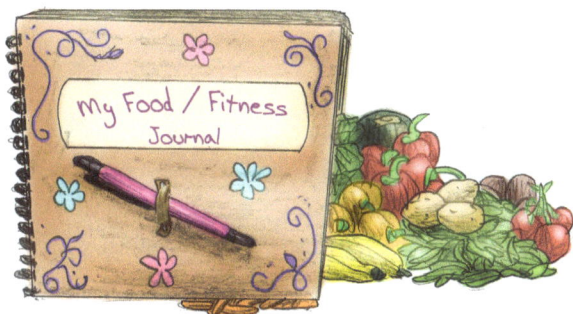

Your Fitness Journal

Here are some ideas to help get you started:

☐ Focus on your efforts and progress

☐ Write down inspiring quotes or healthy tips—any-thing that excites you!

☐ Make an inspiring collage, either in your journal or on a separate vision board that you can hang up and view often. Here are some ideas for your vision board/collage:

  ☐ Cut out motivating quotes, positive words, or af-firmations that inspire you.

  ☐ If your goal is to eat clean and healthy, add pic-tures of clean foods that inspire you to eat healthy.

  ☐ Take full body pictures of yourself – front, back, and side view. Date the pictures and place them on your vision board. In the past I would take full body pictures of myself every six to eight weeks. It's a fun way of tracking progress and staying motivated.

  ☐ If your goal is to run a 5k or participate in a mar-athon, bike-a-thon, or triathlon, cut out pictures of runners, swimmers, and bikers and add them to your board with some positive affirmations, quotes, or words.

☐ Keep an exercise and food log every day. This can also be done either inside or outside of your fitness journal. Personally, I choose to use a separate weekly planner and divide it into two columns. One side is to track my workout, and the other is to track my food. I use a green pen for my workouts and a blue pen for my food log to help keep them separate, but you can use whatever method works best for you.

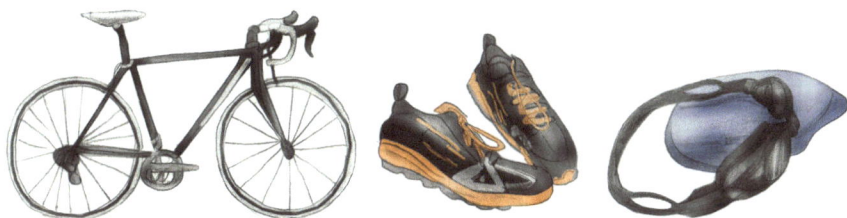

Exercise and Food Log: Keeping Yourself Accountable

When keeping track of your fitness workouts and your meals, you're not only giving yourself a clearer understanding of how you're doing; you're also holding yourself accountable. By holding yourself accountable, you are empowering yourself with awareness. If you come to realize that certain foods taste really great but don't make your body feel so great, it is your empowering decision as to whether or not you want to keep eating these foods. If you find that you've been pushing yourself too hard in your cardio, it is in your hands as to whether or not you'll cut back on your routine.

In building your awareness, you may want to track your training sessions and meals in greater detail, and that's wonderful! You may want to include some detailed information, such as:

For exercise:

☐ Number of sets and repetitions

☐ Warm-up and cool-down routines.

☐ Cardio: note your target heart rate and how you felt before, during, and/or after your workout

☐ Note your progress and personal records

For food:

☐ Record all meals, snacks, and beverages, including as many ingredients as possible

☐ Record the amount of water you take in daily, keeping it in its own category

☐ Note your reaction to certain foods/ingredients, whether it be bodily or emotional

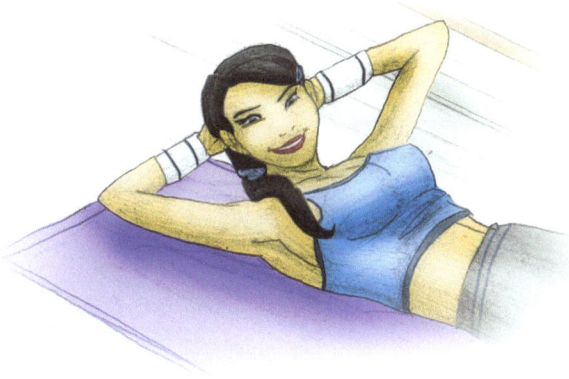

25 Ways to Stay Motivated While Getting Fit and Healthy

When you make the decision to get healthy and fit by beginning a diet and exercise program, it can be difficult to keep yourself motivated—that is, if you don't know all the tips and tricks. One of the biggest secrets is that happy people tend to be more motivated, so you'll find a more in-depth guide to what you've already learned in these 25 inspirational tips that will keep you motivated to reach your fitness goals!

1. **Think healthy lifestyle, healthy living.** You should definitely be excited about the prospect of losing weight. However, what's more exciting than your new outer appearance is just how amazing you can feel about yourself while making drastic lifestyle changes. Living a healthy lifestyle is inspiring and empowering,

which means that *you* can be inspiring and empowering to others! As you learn how to respect, honor, and love your body while on your fitness journey, it's your discoveries, epiphanies, and inner changes that will keep you motivated. All of these will merely be reflected by your new outer appearance—a small perk, when all is said and done.

2. **Set reachable and reasonable goals.** Don't set yourself up for failure by saying that you want to lose 30 lbs. in two-weeks. Miracles do happen; however, when it comes to weight loss, you want to release the weight over a reasonable amount of time. Not only is this far healthier, but you're also going to feel great by actually accomplishing what you've set out to do! For example, you could set a goal to lose 10 lbs. in two weeks or 20 lbs. in one month.

3. **Be accountable.** Write down your goals, say them out loud, or tell them to a friend. By making your goals concrete, in some form or another, you are far less likely to back out on them. Plus, when you write out your desires or say them out loud, you may surprise yourself with it is you really want in life!

4. **Toss out the junk food from your cupboards, refrigerator, and secret stashes—yea, I know about those secret stashes.** Remember when Grandma used to grow sodium aluminosilicate in the garden? Oh...you don't? If you can't pronounce the ingredients on your food labels, there's a good chance that

you don't want them in your body. While it's okay to indulge once in a while, don't keep tempting foods in the house. Treat yourself out to dinner or to a snack every once in while, but having these foods in your house is making them a part of you and your lifestyle, which is exactly what you don't want. The majority of the appeal is in the convenience and the marketing anyways. After you've been eating nutrient rich foods for some time, you may actually find that you don't even *like* this other "food" any more!

5. **Cook your own meals.** Don't groan. Cooking can be fun and easy! Believe it or not, you can make a delicious, nutrient rich meal in less than 30 minutes. You can also save time by cooking in bulk and bringing the leftovers for lunch the next day, or by having your family join in and help out. Cooking is an amazing stress-reliever and creative outlet and can be a great reward to yourself at the end of your work day. In addition, being a part of the full process makes you appreciate your food so much more! Make your meals a labor of love, and allow yourself to enjoy them as such.

6. **Use color psychology.** The color blue is known as an honest, trusting, calming, and loyal color, but did you know that it's also considered an appetite suppressant? So is the color green![48] By eating on blue or green dinner plates, or by eating in a blue or green dining room/kitchen, you can actually psychologically help to curb your appetite! Doesn't painting the

kitchen sound like an awesome way to get exercise *and* change your eating habits?

7. **Celebrate milestones.** When you lose 5, 10, or 15 pounds, celebrate it! Treat yourself to a spa day or a movie. Have a well-balanced meal with friends and family. Congratulate yourself for reaching your small goals, and celebrate the new you!

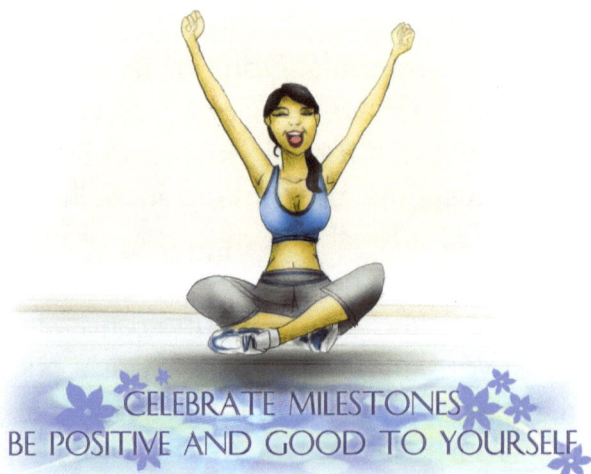

CELEBRATE MILESTONES
BE POSITIVE AND GOOD TO YOURSELF

8. **Don't be too hard on yourself.** Everyone has good days and bad days. You may not reach your goals every day or every week, but that's okay—this happens to everyone. Shake it off and keep moving forward on your journey. Keep a positive attitude and always get back to your routine—whatever it is that works best for you.

9. **Get rid of your "all or nothing" attitude.** Here's a secret: no one is perfect. You may strive to be perfect, and that's wonderful. But unfortunately, neither you nor I are perfect. Having an "all or nothing" attitude will set you up for disappointment. And believe it or not, having this mentality actually stems from the *fear* that you can't do it. *You* know you can, and *I* know you can. Commit to living a fit and healthy lifestyle 100 percent, and give it your *all*! If you slip up here and there, it's not the end of the world, and you are still AMAZING for putting in all your hard work!

10. **Sleep.** Getting at least eight hours of sleep will do your body, mind, and soul good. You may be thinking, "I can't get eight hours of sleep a night!" Well, I am here to tell you that you can, and you will! If it's important to you, you'll make time. Bottom line.

11. **Motivate** *yourself!* Relying on others to be your cheerleader isn't a good idea. Not only do others tend to be unreliable in fulfilling your every desire, but you are also doing yourself a *huge* disservice by seeking motivation in others. You will actually *lose* self-confidence by relying on others for affirmations that you can and should be giving to *yourself*! Be your own cheerleader and root for YOU!

12. **Keep a food journal.** Writing down what you eat throughout the day will help you actually see all that you're consuming. All of those snacks, alcoholic

beverages, and sweet beverages that we wouldn't think of otherwise can really add up! When you write it all down, it's almost like you're telling on yourself (and you'll know if you haven't written everything). Even if you're the only one who sees what you write, you'll still want to be proud of what you record in your journal. Keeping a food journal is, by far, one of the best self-motivators for eating healthy.

13. **Get rid of your "fat" clothes.** Once you begin to lose weight, donate your old clothes. Get rid of them so that you don't have larger clothing hanging around, you know, just in case. This is a long-term change, and that weight is staying off for good! Plus, giving away your old clothes because they don't *fit* and more…feels *amazing!*

14. **Download some new music.** There's nothing more motivating or inspiring sometimes than hearing new music. Exchange playlists with a friend! Have fun with it and start moving to the beat!

15. **Surround yourself with people who'll support you.** Like it or not, your family and friends may not support the fact that you want to get fit and healthy. The simple truth is that not everyone is motivated enough him- or herself to do what you're doing, and that's it—it's nothing to be taken personally. However, it is important to have people around you who *are* supportive—and they are out there! All you have to do is give what you want to receive and set the intention

to attract supportive people into your life. Before you know it, you'll be seeing new smiling faces all around you!

16. **Join a support group.** Find a group that's positive and fun! Some groups can concentrate a great deal on the negative aspects of the past, which can be great for helping to relieve some more deep-seated issues. However, staying in such groups can keep you wallowing in self-pity, which can be the opposite of motivating. Find a group with energy and positivity to help motivate you on your journey!

17. **List the reasons "why" you want to lose weight and get healthy.** Look at your list from time to time to keep you remembering your personal motivations. The deeper and more personal the reasons, the deeper your connection will be, and the more you will want to fulfill these deep desires.

18. **Focus on the positives in your life.** When you act positively, you attract positivity. The same happens with the opposite. When you think and act negatively, you also attract negativity—and nobody wants that. Any energy that you want to receive must be genuinely given, so if you want love, you must give love. There will be days in which feeling positive will be easy, and you'll feel wonderful as you absolutely radiate positivity! Then, you'll likely have some difficult days. And that's okay! You don't have to feel like a superhero every day, and you certainly don't want

to fake your emotions. However, you should always remember to lead with a positive attitude, no matter what your daily obstacles may be.

19. **A change of scenery is good.** This may be a home workout program, but that doesn't mean staying in your house all day. Breathe some fresh air into your lungs! Go to a park to meditate, or take a walk and maybe meet someone new! Go out to a local café, take an interesting class, or volunteer! Your options are endless, especially when you get creative.

20. **Replace negative self-talk with positive self-talk.** We already covered general positivity, but you must also understand the crucial importance of ridding yourself of negative self-talk. There's a great deal of chatter that goes on in our brains, of which many of us are not even aware. Make it a goal to become aware of what it is you say to yourself. If you don't like what you hear, then for the sake of your own healing and motivation, you must start making a change. Start training yourself to speak and think positively about yourself. If you want to believe in yourself, then you will with practice. We've all been to a party and had a long chat with someone about all the reasons why he or she is *not* doing what s/he wants to be doing, or why s/he *wishes* that s/he were doing something that s/he is not—it's this kind of talk that's not serving anyone. Be the positive light at a party, and be this same positive light within yourself.

21. **Toss out the words I CAN'T.** Yes, you can! The words, "I can't," carry a powerful affirmation equivalent with, "I give up," and, "I'm not worth it." Start replacing, "I can't," with, "I can!" You'll be amazed by just how much you can accomplish.

22. **Start your day early.** Just because you've gotten out of bed and shoveled a spoonful of sustenance into your body before rushing out the door, doesn't mean that you're really awake or ready to start your day. Give yourself some time in the morning to really wake up and feel ready to start your day. There's nothing like giving yourself time to move at your own pace or to just spend some quality alone time. When you start your day early with a full body workout, yoga, meditation, or something that you do just for your-self, you will start out feeling energized, refreshed, excited, and renewed. You'll start out feeling completely fulfilled before you even start your work day, which will help clear your mind for the rest of the day in addition to helping you sleep better at night.

23. **Practice an attitude of gratitude.** Everyone, no matter who he or she might be, has something for which to be grateful, and practicing gratitude can be extremely motivating. If you simply start by being grateful for your life, this is simple but strong. You could die tomorrow, but you're alive RIGHT NOW! What are you most motivated to do in these crucial hours that could possibly be your last?

24. **Read success stories.** Read books, read articles, watch documentaries—you name it! Get inspired by others who have traveled down your path (or at least a path that seems similar and intriguing to you). Find role models and nutrition facts that inspire you. There is so much information in this world and so much proof that you are not alone!

25. **Believe in YOU!** Believe in your strength and ability. Believe in your willpower and your endurance. Have faith in yourself, and know that you are worth it! Everyone deserves to be healthy and happy, and everyone deserves to feel great in his or her own skin. You are no exception!

Stay Motivated, Stay on Your Fit and Healthy Journey

Your fitness journey may not be easy at first, and it may not be easy every step of the way. However, it will become easier as time goes on, and using the tips above to help you along the way will help to make your journey fun and adventure filled.

Just remember, this is not a race. It's a lifestyle change—one that's better for you, your family, your friends, and all others around you. I know that I may have mentioned this once or twice before, but it's important to *believe in yourself.* By doing this, you are not only helping others to believe in you, but also to believe in themselves. You are sheer inspiration, you saucy fitness queen! Keep up the good work!

STAYING FIT WHILE TRAVELING

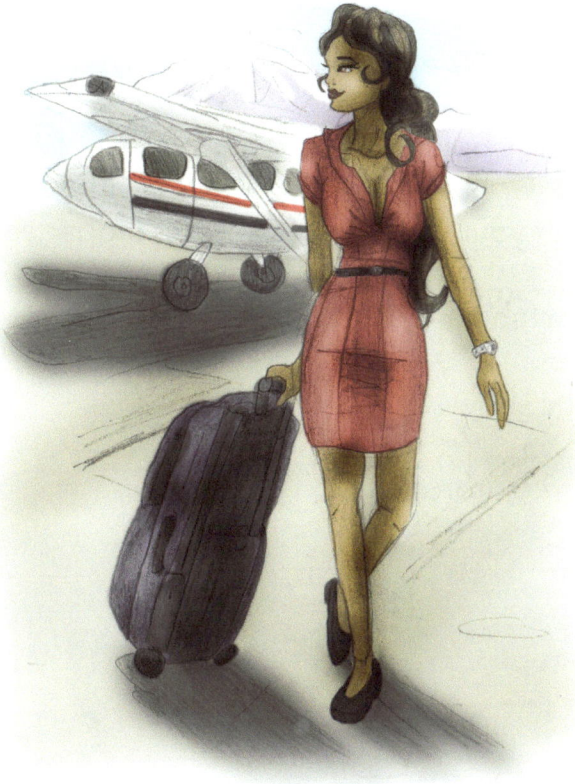

WHEN YOU TRAVEL, YOU MIGHT think that you can't work out, because you don't have your workout equipment with you. Luckily, most hotels, resorts, motels, etc. have fitness centers on site. But what happens if you stay at a bed and breakfast? What about a hostel? How about a campground? What about a cabin? Heck, maybe you just don't want to work out at a fitness center. The good news is that you *can* work out when you travel, because you'll have the greatest tool kit with you: you guessed it, the *Click it to Rip it* app and eBook! The following tips are here to keep you fit and healthy, no matter your location.

What to Pack in Your Suitcase or Carry-On Luggage

The checklist below will give you everything you need and more to work out while traveling without taking up much space in your suitcase or carry-on luggage:

- ☐ Comfortable workout clothes

- ☐ Athletic shoes

- ☐ Heart monitor

- ☐ Weight bands

- ☐ Jump rope

How to Stay Fit While You Travel – With Travel Workout Equipment

Below are ways for you to get an amazing cardio workout with minimal workout equipment.

Step 1 – Jump rope

After you've changed into your workout clothes and laced up your sneakers, grab your jump rope and find your workout space, whether it be indoors our outdoors.

> **Tip:** Don't forget to wear your heart monitor so you can track your beats per minute.

Jump rope for a count of 100. Or, start slow by doing three sets of ten repetitions.

Step 2 – Weight bands

Warm up your body by doing some stretching exercises, and then grab your weight bands and start working those muscles! Stand, holding the middle of the band beneath your feet. Hold the handles on either, pulling your arms up towards your chest, and give yourself a good bicep workout! Do three sets of ten repetitions with your weight bands.

How to Stay Fit While You Travel – Without Travel Workout Equipment

Of course, you can stay fit while you travel *without* packing a single piece of workout equipment in your carry-on or suitcase. Below are some cardio exercises you can do from the comfort of your hotel/motel room, cabin, campground, RV, etc.

Step 1 – March to it

Change into your workout clothes and put on your athletic shoes. Crank up your favorite music, because it will help you get into the marching zone.

Find a comfortable spot in your room or outside and start marching in place. Get your knees up high, as if you're trying to touch your chin with your knees. Do this for about five to ten minutes at a time, and rest at 30-second intervals in between marching. You can also march for any smaller time interval, such as one minute, and rest for 30 seconds in between.

When you march in place, you work your thighs, hips, abdominals, and buttocks. Once again, work to really lift your knees, but only lift as high as waist level. March in place 3-4 times per day and you'll continue to burn calories while you travel.

Step 2 – Calisthenics

You can do other cardio exercises such as jumping jacks, jogging in place (just like marching in place), sit-ups, push-ups, "invisible" jump rope, waist twists, windmills, and crunches. Do a combination of these exercises for about 20 minutes to 30 minutes once, twice, or three times a day. Focus on your breath, quality, and form. Again, you can rest for thirty seconds between sets.

Step 3 – Cross-country ski anytime of the year

After you have changed into your workout clothes and put on your shoes, you're ready to begin cross-country skiing, no poles or snow required.

- ☐ Stand with your feet shoulder width apart and put your left foot in front of your right foot, about two to three feet.

- ☐ With a quick jump, switch the position of your feet so your right foot is now in front of your left foot (in a way that mimics the motion of cross-country skiing). Your left arm should be extended in front like you're holding a ski pole.

- ☐ Now, switch back. Your left foot should be in front of your right foot. Your right arm should be extended in front like you're holding a ski pole.

Do this for one minute and increase your time as you get comfortable and stronger. The motion can take practice, but once you get used to it, you'll have a blast!

HEALTHY LIVING | HEALTHY LIFESTYLE

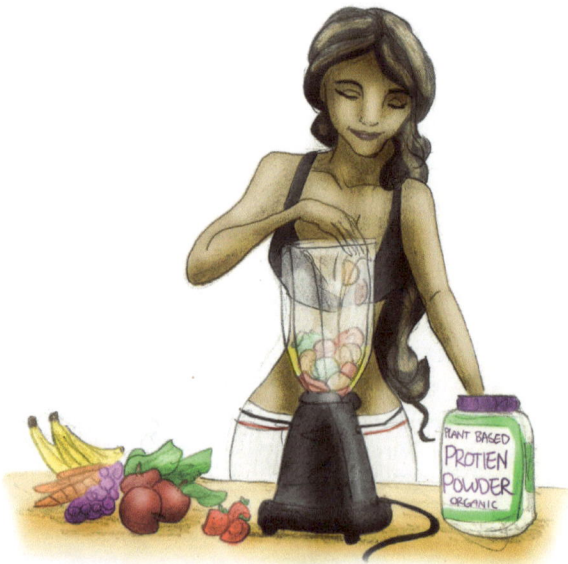

LIVING A HEALTHY LIFESTYLE IS not difficult if you truly want to get fit and stay fit for the rest of your life. The changes you make today can and will be everlasting, if you're willing to commit to keeping these changes and growing (or shrinking, depending on your perspective) with these changes. So, are you ready for healthy living and a healthy lifestyle? If you shouted, *"Yes!"* sit back and keep reading because you're in for a real treat. Don't worry; this one won't add inches to your hips, abdominals, thighs, or buttocks.

Nutrition Motivation

Regular exercise is one component to starting your weight loss. Another is proper nutrition. When you combine exercise with good nutrition, you jump start your weight loss (and can maintain it) in addition to reducing the stress you put on your body, especially your heart.

As you begin listening to your body, you'll realize that it can tell you exactly what it likes and what it doesn't like. When a healthy lifestyle is important to you, and when you begin to pick up on these messages from your body, your mind will begin to choose the foods that your body enjoys, rather than solely what your taste buds enjoy. Eating a healthy, balanced, and nutrient rich diet every day can be extremely simple in this way.

Being your personal trainer and guide, I'm going to give you some tips from my personal diet to help get you started. What follows are some tasty tips for eating cleanly, organically, and what's right for your body. As a bonus, I've also included some of my personal favorite recipes!

Ready? Let's go!

My Nutrition and Lifestyle

In order to help you gain perspective and insight on your own journey, I've chosen to share with you my personal nutrition and lifestyle journey:

As long as I can remember, I have always had digestive issues. As a child, I was never tested for food intolerances, because my digestive issues simply weren't thought of in such a way. I had difficulty producing bowel movements, which my parents treated with over the counter laxatives. At the age of six, while living in Brisbane, Australia, I was hospitalized due to a constipation that was so severe, the doctors wanted to do surgery. Even then, no one recommended that I be tested for allergies—it just wasn't the mindset at the time.

For years, I experienced abdominal pain, cramping, bloating, constipation, and other embarrassing and painful symptoms. Being that my heritage is European (my father Czechoslovakian and my mother Romanian), meat was a huge part of my diet growing up and continued to remain so until 2012, when my digestive issues worsened. After being diagnosed by a gastrologist with irritable bowel syndrome (IBS), I began to make some serious diet changes. For the first time in my life, I began treating the causes instead of the symptoms. I listened to my body and kept a food log of my meals, noting any reactions to the foods I ate. It was a process of elimination that led me to find that I had reactions to meat, dairy, and other insoluble fiber foods.

Even though I was working hard at listening to my body and working on the process of elimination, I still wasn't completely certain of what I could and couldn't eat. This meant that I still had flare-ups, and there was still pain. At times, the pain was so bad that it brought tears to my eyes. So, I decided to go back to the gastrologist and have my very first food intolerance testing. I was excited by the prospect of finally and definitively knowing the causes of my symptoms. The test was performed in four parts: glucose test, fructose test, lactose test, and Mediator Release Test. I had blood my drawn and promptly sent to a lab. When the results came back two weeks later, I received a book of foods to which my body had a reaction. This information confirmed my personal experiment results and then some, which was a major breakthrough for me!

I am a huge believer in staying prescription medication free. However, my first two specialists highly suggested this expensive medication that would cost me 100 to 200 dollars per month. One of them told me that I just had to learn to live with it. Neither of these were suitable options for me, so I went my own route. I started eating a vegan and gluten free diet and now avoid the foods to which I have intolerances. I have never felt better!

After making my decision, I went to see my nutritionist in order to make sure I wasn't missing any nutrients in my diet. We sat down together and created new meal plans for me. I now eat a nutrient rich, well balanced, and tasty diet without feeling the pain caused by unnecessary added foods.

Through my own journey, I am able to share how you too can feel amazing and stay healthy. Some of you may have similar digestive issues, and some of you may not. My hope is to inspire, inform, and incite both those who do and those who do not struggle with IBS, and to make all of my information clear and accessible.

I encourage every woman to back up her diet and life-style with regular check ups performed by a doctor and to nourish her body with clean food—to replace refined, processed, and toxic food with clean meals, lean proteins, complex carbohydrates, and healthy fats.

Irritable Bowel Syndrome (IBS)

If you have experienced severe abdominal pain, cramp-ing, bloating, stomach distension, gas, diarrhea, and/or constipation for an extended period of time, or if you have been diagnosed with IBS, I highly recommend speaking with your doctor about receiving a Mediator Release Test (MRT). There can be a deeper cause than IBS to your pain, and you don't just have to "live with it." Let's enjoy life pain free!

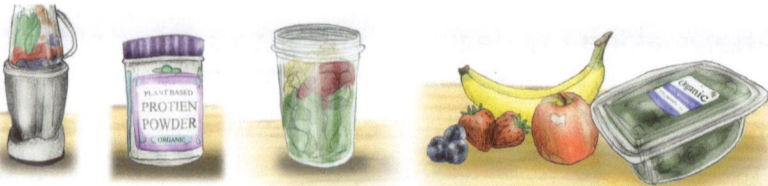

Should You Become a Vegan?

There are many reasons why people choose to eat a vegetarian, vegan, raw, and/or gluten free diet, but this is a personal decision. This is also a decision that can evolve and change over time. I don't believe that there is any one diet that is suitable for everyone or even suitable for a lifetime—everyone is different. The most important thing to remember is to listen to your body as you eat. Being a vegan doesn't necessarily mean being healthy. There are many vegans who actually *gain* weight after making the switch, because once they hear that things like Oreos are vegan— yea, you heard me—they go to flippin' town!

If you're still curious about whether or not Oreos are really vegan, you can read the label yourself! One thing about a vegan and/or gluten free lifestyle is that you'll find yourself reading all of your food labels. If, however, you're reading the ingredient labels for health reasons, you will quickly come to see just how unappealing foods with sugar or high fructose corn syrup as their first ingredients can be. Eating a vegan diet helps you think about what it is you're really putting into your body, which is very important and very beneficial to someone seeking to lose weight.

Believe it or not, it is possible to get all the nutrients you need from a plant-based diet, and there are many health benefits that accompany such a diet. You just need to make sure that your diet is well planed and well balanced. Your balanced plant-based diet should include whole grains, heart-healthy fats, protein, veggies, and fruit. In addition to those, I personally take an algae based Omega 3 multivitamin and hair/nail supplements. All of my vitamins are organic.

Note: Vitamins should be person specific, as everyone has different needs.

Once again, this is a personal decision, and everyone is different. Due to different illnesses, conditions, diseases, and allergies, people can be restricted from eating a great deal of foods. If you already have severe food restrictions, adding the restrictions of a vegetarian/vegan/raw/gluten free diet may cause you to miss out on needed nutrients and could potentially put your health at risk. Again, please speak with your doctor and nutritionist, because they can help guide you to make the right decisions for your body.

If you find out that the vegan or vegetarian lifestyle isn't for you, then just add in or substitute what you do eat with the diet that follows. When eating meat, eat lean, organic meats. In addition, meat from a cow should be grass-fed. Meat is a good source of protein, and it's important to have twenty grams of protein at each of five to six small meals a day to help you lose weight. Whether you eat meat or not, you need protein.

Protein and the Vegan Lifestyle

"How do you get your protein?" is always the main question posed to vegans and vegetarians. The truth of the matter is that there are *many* ways to get protein. The following list can be your go-to-guide for implementing enough protein into your diet:

- ☐ Vegetables (particularly leafy greens and legumes)

- ☐ Nuts (and nut butters like peanut, almond, and cashew butters)

- ☐ Seeds (sesame, sunflower, poppy, hemp, chia, etc.)

- ☐ Beans (black, red, navy, white, soy, garbanzo, etc.)

- ☐ Non-dairy milk (coconut, rice, almond, hemp, soy, etc.—try making your own to cut down on additives and cost!)

- ☐ Quinoa

- ☐ Tempeh

- ☐ Tofu

- ☐ Protein shakes

- ☐ And many more!

Protein shakes are one of my favorite protein supplements, because they are great for people who work out. I use organic, plant based protein powder to create my shakes. I also like to play around with adding different natural healing elements to my shakes, such as turmeric powder, chia seeds, and other plant-based healers. Then, I add a banana for sweetness. The main protein powder I use is the Garden of Life Raw Protein®, but I also like to change things up every once in a while. Whenever I look at purchasing a product, I always check the ingredients to make sure that everything is vegan and organic. I also do my research to make sure that the brand uses good practices. Protein shakes are safe for people who are healthy and fit and are mostly used by athletes; you can choose to drink one after you've finished your workout instead of making a meal.[49] Just keep in mind that protein shakes are not food replacements and cannot be substituted as the majority of your meals. I usually have one in the morning and/or pre-workout.

I understand the vital importance of protein to my diet, which is why I incorporate it into every meal. A good amount of protein helps to burn fat and builds muscle when combined with a workout plan. Our bodies also use the proteins in our diet to maintain tissue and build new cells.

Sample Meal Plan

Below is a sample of my personal meal plan for one day:

7:00 a.m. – Gluten free oatmeal, strawberries with walnuts, and grapefruit on the side.

10:00 a.m. – Lara Bar (homemade) and banana.

1:00 p.m. – Salad: spinach, quinoa, brown rice, garbanzo beans, and tomatoes with safflower oil and salt.

4:00 p.m. – Protein Shake: Garden of Life Raw Protein powder (plant based), chia seeds, strawberries, banana, spinach, and water.

7:00 p.m. – Beans (organic, BPA free pinto, black, or garbanzo beans, Eden brand), brown rice, organic Maitake mushrooms, safflower oil, and salt.

10:00 p.m. – Avocado

Calories

Personal trainers are often asked, "How many calories should I eat?" This is a great question to ask, because the answer varies from woman to woman.

Below are calculators based on the Harris-Benedict formula to help you figure out how many calories you need. For example, I work out four days a week and need to consume 1,638 calories to maintain my weight. Figure out the amount of calories you need in your daily diet so that you can eat a healthy and accurate amount for your body.

Basal Metabolic Rate (BMR)50

Women: BMR = 655 + (4.35 x weight in pounds) + (4.7 x height in inches) - (4.7 x age in years)

Men: BMR = 66 + (6.23 x weight in pounds) + (12.7 x height in inches) - (6.8 x age in years)

Active Metabolic Rate (AMR)51

Calculate your AMR by using your BMR and estimating your current level of activity. Activity levels and calculations are as follows:

☐ Sedentary (little or no exercise) = BMR x 1.2

☐ Lightly active (light exercise/work 1-3 days per week) = BMR x 1.375

☐ Moderately active (moderate exercise/work 3-5 days per week) = BMR x 1.55

☐ Very active (hard exercise/work 6-7 days a week) = BMR x 1.725

☐ Extra active (very hard exercise/work 6-7 days a week) = BMR x 1.9

After you've calculated the number of calories (AMR) for your body, you'll be able to formulate a nutrition plan that works for you. You can consult with your doctor or nutritionist for help creating your meal plans. To lose weight, increase your physical activity, or decrease the number of calories you consume each day.

Hint: Decrease your calorie intake by 500 calories every day and you'll lose about one pound each week. Make sure your calorie intake is not LESS than 1,200 calories.

Don't go on a crash diet because they're not safe or effective.

Food and Drink

Water

Water is extremely important to a healthy lifestyle. The standard advice is to drink eight cups every day; however, you should aim for about 9 cups (2.2 liters) daily. You'll need to drink more water during the warmer months, or if you exercise on a regular basis. If you don't like drinking water, add lemon or cucumbers to give it some flavor.

Carbs

You don't have to give up carbs! Complex carbs are good for you and are crucial to your daily energy levels. They're found in whole foods like brown rice, potatoes, oatmeal, whole barley, and even fruits and vegetables—spinach, apples, asparagus, strawberries, grapefruit, and more. Even though complex carbs are good for you, portion control is still important.

Simple carbohydrates are the ones you want to avoid, especially if you want to lose weight. They are broken down quickly into glucose, which makes up glycogen. Body cells can only store a limited amount of glycogen, and taking in too many simple carbohydrates may contribute to body fat stores. The simple carbs you want to avoid are cake, candy, refined sugar, fruit juice, soda, honey, milk, corn syrup, jam, foods baked with white flour, and the list goes on.

Processed Foods

Avoid processed foods, because they have been altered from their natural state for convenience. Packaged foods filled with strong, addicting flavors, that also have loads of ingredients are harmful to your body. People on a highly processed-based diet run the risk of obesity, heart disease, and even cancer (caused by some of the synthetic chemicals used in the processed food industry known to have carcinogenic properties).

Instead of buying a package of hummus, for example, try making it yourself out of whole foods. You'll be surprised at how fresh and delicious it tastes compared to the processed kind. The best part is that your hummus will have only fresh ingredients, keeping the unnecessary, added ingredients out of your body.

Soda

If you drink soda or diet soda, you may want to reconsider. Your diet soda has shown itself to be packed with sugar and cause obesity,[52] kidney trouble, tooth decay, and weakening of the bones[53]; it messes with your metabolism and causes cell damage and reproductive issues. The Aspartame in diet soda raises blood glucose levels, and when your liver encounters too much glucose, the excess converts to body fat. Even though the FDA approved aspartame, there have been ninety-two acknowledged different symptoms caused by aspartame that result in indigestion.

Alcohol

Alcohol is very high in calories and should be taken in sparingly. Some people choose to be completely alcohol free, which has extreme health benefits. However, this is a personal choice. When you drink alcohol, try to avoid the sweeter beverages, and count each glass as part of your caloric intake.

Coffee

For those of you who are coffee drinkers, it is recommended by doctors that you have no more than two five-ounce cups per day. It's also best to drink organic coffee without sugar and without aspartame or powdered creamers.

Though we don't treat it as such, caffeine is a drug to which there are many side effects. It affects nearly every organ, which includes your skin and your nervous system. There is no nutritional value in drinking coffee. For me and for my IBS, coffee causes more pain than pleasure, and I choose to avoid it as much as possible.

Chocolate

Did you know that eating small amounts of dark chocolate two to three times each week could lower your blood pressure? Studies have shown that dark chocolate can improve blood flow, may help prevent heart disease (hardening of the arteries),[54] protect the skin, and improve your mood. Just make sure the dark chocolate is made organically and by a trusted brand. Check the ingredients to make sure that they are minimal. The fewer the ingredients on the label, the healthier the chocolate will be. Plus, once you get out of the Hershey's realm, you'll see just how little real cocoa you need satisfy you—small amounts two to three times a week, to be precise!

Cheat Day

Cheat days keep your body guessing and boost your metabolism. Having one cheat day a week is good, especially when you're restricting calories and sticking to a clean eating plan the rest of the week. I see my cheat day as my mental break from dieting and training. On my cheat day, I don't journal anything, and I make this day my well deserved day off to just relax. I don't eat much more on my cheat days, because I've gotten used to my healthy lifestyle and don't like the feeling of overeating. However, I don't pass judgment on myself for a little extra indulgence. I also don't feel pressured to make the most out of my cheat day if I'm really just not in the mood for something super sweet or savory that day (it happens). If I've got my mind on something, I'll appreciate it much more when my next cheat day rolls around.

If you are a diabetic or have digestive or other health issues, you must keep this in mind when choosing your "cheat" food. If you want to eat something you can't have, don't have it. Your body and your health is always more important than a temporary sensation. Cheat with foods that you *can* have, and you'll appreciate them just as much.

Eating Organic Foods

Organic farmers grow and process agriculture products by maintaining and replenishing the soil's fertility naturally, without the use of pesticides and toxic fertilizers. Organic food may cost you more in the grocery store due to the additional labor involved in the organic process, but the fact that you are keeping literal poison out of your body is well worth it. Foods are meant to be nourishing, not toxic.

Cut down on your organic costs by growing a few things yourself! Getting in touch with the growing process is not only therapeutic, but also a great way to help you think about where your food comes from. Another way to eat locally and organically is by shopping at a farmer's market or by joining a CSA (Community Supported Agriculture). The idea behind a CSA is that you (the community) support a local farm by paying for the upcoming season's crop production. You buy a share or a membership in exchange for a box of produce, available for you and your family each week of the farming season.

If you are a meat and/or dairy consumer, then you should *definitely* be buying organic products. When cows are being fed hormones, such as rBGH, you too are consuming these hormones in your beef and your milk. We have yet to know the effects of such hormones, which is less than settling to any conscious consumer. The most nutritious and safest bet for you and your family is to eat as many organic and non-GMO (Genetically Modified Organism) foods as possible.

Yes, grocery shopping will take a little extra time at first, but once you know what to look for, your shopping experience will become much quicker again. However, your shopping experience will be forever changed. Being a conscious consumer is empowering, and it makes every single action one of difference.

Tip: Shop the outside aisles, because this is where you'll find more of what you're looking for. The inner aisles are all of the pre-packaged and processed foods, of which you'll want far less.

Eating for Your Body

It's important to understand what foods are best for your body. Remember, your body is different from the body of your sister, best friend, mom, aunt, etc. Make an appointment and speak with a nutritionist about putting together a plan that works for your body. If you're a diabetic or have high blood pressure or irritable bowel syndrome (IBS), you MUST find out what foods are right for your body. Otherwise, you could experience pain and discomfort for the rest of your life. And worse, you could be put on medication for the rest of your life. If you can make these changes for yourself, it's possible to live life pain and medication free!

So often, we rush from day to day, thinking about everything but our body—one of our most important assets in life. Listen to your body, and respect your body--you've only got one with which to live in this lifetime. Your stomach won't always do back flips at the end of an incompatible meal to tell you that something is going wrong (thought you should definitely know that something is wrong when your stomach is doing such acrobatic tricks). Sometimes, our bodies react in the very smallest subtleties, such as inflammation in the joints or mild chest pains, to let us know what our bodies could truly do without. Listen deeply to your body, and respond as necessary. Do some experiments of your own, and talk to your doctor or nutritionist to find out more.

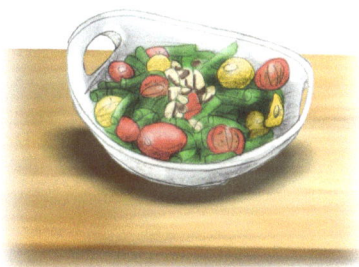

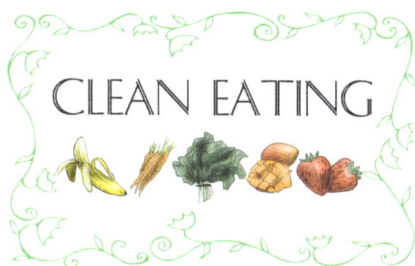

Clean Eating

When it comes to losing fat, it's important that you make good eating choices and snack smart. This takes a good amount of will power and self-control, but you can do it!

There are many delicious, clean food choices out there, and you can make the switch to clean eating without sacrificing the taste and enjoyment of other foods.

You may be thinking to yourself, "Anna, how can I switch to clean eating when I crave certain foods like potato chips all the time?" That's easy. Whenever I am fixating on a bad snack, I first check to see whether or not I'm actually hungry—most of the time, a craving is just a desire for the sensation of eating. Whether I'm hungry or not (but especially if I'm not hungry), I pour myself a glass of water instead. If I'm still hungry or still can't seem to kick my craving, I go to my pantry or my refrigerator and look at my alternative snacks. There are many easy options to throw together quickly, like organic fruit and natural peanut butter. But when I just can't seem to kick the craving, I turn to one of my favorite alternative snacks: plain-aired popcorn with some olive oil, sea salt, pepper, and/or other seasonings. Yummy! Since making the change to eating cleaner foods, I don't feel like I'm missing out on the potato chips any more.

Clean eating is a lifestyle. It means that you no longer put junk foods into your body. You pay attention to the menu when you dine out. You make conscious food choices by reading labels when you go grocery shopping, and you keep a food journal to track the foods that don't agree with YOUR body.

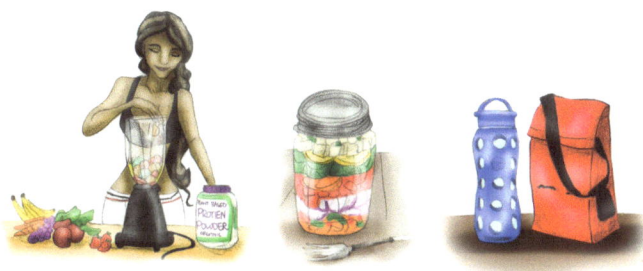

How Do You Eat When You Are Super Busy?

You're probably thinking, "Anna, I am so busy--I'm a wife and a mom, and I work full-time. I don't have time to even think about eating cleaner foods!"

When you're super busy, it's easy to get overwhelmed. However, taking the time to sit down and write it out, paradoxically, helps cut down on your time and stress. I plan my meals ahead of time by writing them down. Once I've written down some fun food ideas and some successful meals, it's easy to plan my meals and to reuse the meal plans that have worked in the past. I don't like to skip meals, and knowing that my work schedule is very hectic, I never want to risk it. For me, preparing my meals the night before is the best way to avoid this problem or to avoid eating out. I usually bring my little blender to work with me, along with fresh foods that I've prepared in small bags the night before. This way, I can always have a fresh protein shake in the middle of the day.

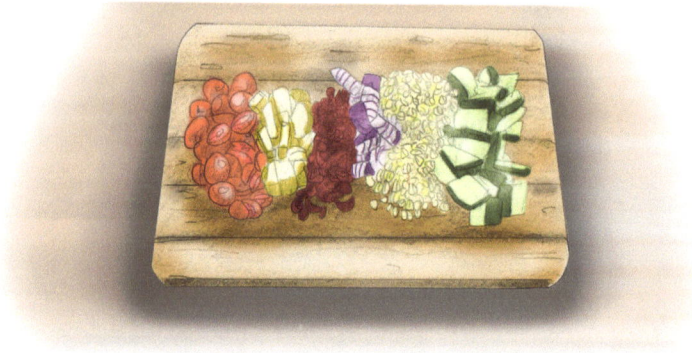

How to Eat Cleanly

You can eat cleanly by doing the following:

☐ Eat 5-6 small meals per day (includes snacks).

☐ Drink more than 8 glasses of water each day.

☐ Read ALL labels when you grocery shop. If you can't pronounce the ingredients on food labels, you probably don't want it in your body. Try to avoid saturated fats, trans fats, and sugar, in addition to processed and refined foods. Watch for cholesterol too. Lastly, be mindful of sugar substitutes, because they may not be as healthy as you think.

☐ Choose organic foods and beverages whenever possible.

☐ Watch your portions. Note: One portion of meat should be no bigger than the size of your palm and no thicker than a stack of cards.

☐ Eat healthy fats, such as nuts/nut butters, avocado, olive oil, flaxseed oil, etc.

☐ Eat those fruits and veggies that are so good and so good for you!

☐ Listen to your body when you eat. If a food doesn't agree with you, write it down and write it out.

☐ Take time to enjoy your meals! Help your digestive system and your taste buds by slowing down the eating process.

☐ Try to eat produce that is seasonal to ensure its freshness and to reduce your carbon footprint.

☐ Eat conscientiously raised meats, such as beef, chicken, fish, turkey, and pork—healthy, organically raised animals produce milk, eggs, and meat that are better for you and that taste better too!

☐ Reduce the amount of alcohol you drink.

☐ Cut back on salt—replace the table salt with sea salt or Himalayan pink salt.

☐ Have a cup of decaffeinated green tea.

☐ Learn how to cook!

Eating cleanly may seem daunting at first, but once you get into the groove of clean eating, it will become second nature. You'll quickly scan through menu items when you dine out and will gain the confidence to ask to have your meal prepared in a healthier way. Before you know it, your family and friends will be commenting in how young and refreshed you look—and of course, they'll all want to know your secret!

Healthy Recipes for a Healthy Lifestyle

Below are some healthy recipes that will keep you full and satisfied. Eat healthy, lose weight, and be happy!

Breakfast

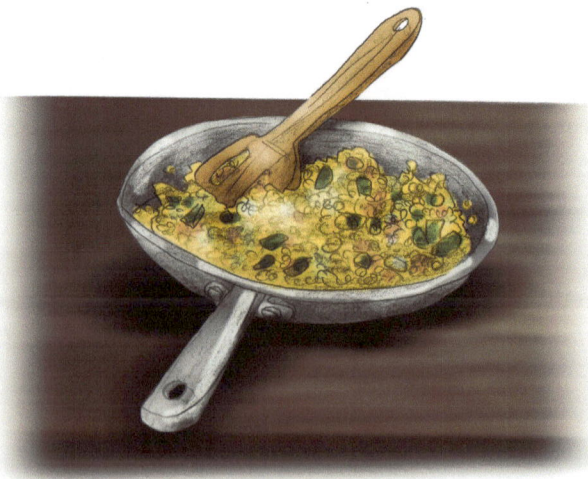

Tofu Scramble (2-4 servings)

1 lb. firm or extra firm tofu, drained, pressed, and crumbled

½ yellow onion, diced

Handful of fresh Maitake mushrooms

2 tablespoons oil

1 teaspoon garlic powder

1 tablespoon nutritional yeast

2 pinches of Kala Namak/black salt (which tends to smell and taste like eggs) or sea salt

½ teaspoon turmeric (this adds color, making your tofu scramble look like scrambled eggs)

Directions

1. Drain the packaged tofu and slightly crumble it with your fork or hand.

2. Sauté onion, mushrooms, and crumbled tofu in oil for 3-5 minutes, stirring regularly.

3. Add the remaining ingredients and cook for 5-7 minutes at medium heat.

4. Keep stirring, add more oil if necessary, and cook until some of the liquid evaporates. Then, remove from heat and serve.

*You may wrap this in a brown rice tortilla with leafy greens to make a breakfast burrito, or just enjoy eating it as is.

*You may also want to add vegetables to your tofu scramble to add extra flavor and nutrients.

Lunch

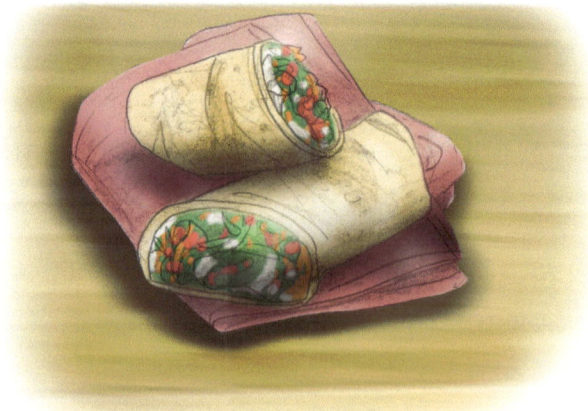

Sandwich Wrap (1 serving)

Homemade hummus spread (see recipe under snack)

Large brown rice tortilla

Handful of shredded carrots

Handful of baby spinach

½ handful of Mung sprout beans

Sprinkle of safflower oil and lemon

3 pinches of sea salt

Avocado slices

Directions

1. Spread the homemade hummus.

2. Add the remaining ingredients in a thinly spread layer.

3. Roll up your wrap tightly. Then, slice into 1-inch thick rounds (optional).

Dinner

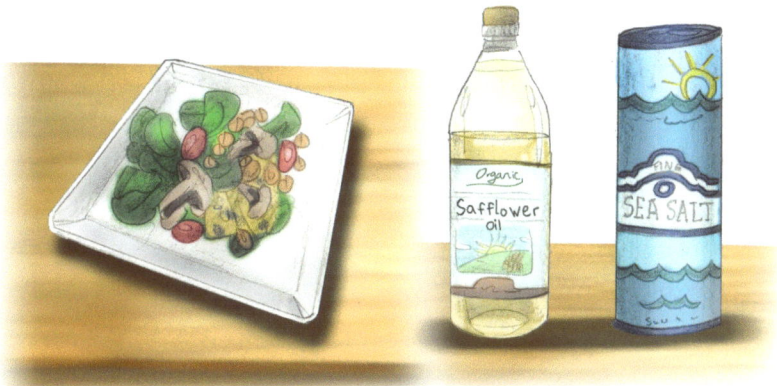

Brown Rice, Quinoa, Bean Salad (6 servings)

1 cup cooked brown rice

½ cup cooked quinoa

1 can (15 ounces) organic beans (any bean of your choice—pinto, black, garbanzo, etc.)

1 cup fresh sliced mushrooms

6 ounces organic baby spinach

1 1/2 cups cherry tomatoes, halved

¼ cup organic safflower oil

sea salt and pepper to taste

Directions

1. Bring quinoa and water to boil in a saucepan. In a separate saucepan, bring brown rice and water to boil. Reduce heat to medium-low, cover, and simmer until quinoa and rice are tender and water has been absorbed. Set aside to cool for 10-15 minutes.

2. Whisk safflower oil, sea salt, and pepper together in a bowl.

3. Combine brown rice, quinoa, garbanzo beans, spinach, mushrooms, and cherry tomatoes together in a bowl. Pour safflower dressing over salad mixture; toss to coat.

Serve immediately or chill in refrigerator.

Snack

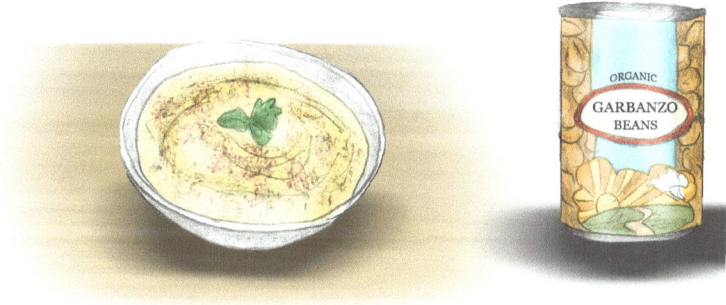

Homemade Hummus

1 can (15 ounce) organic garbanzo beans/chickpeas

1/3 cup tahini

1/3 cup fresh parsley, chopped fine

2 tablespoons fresh lemon juice

3 tablespoons water

1 tablespoon hot sauce or soy sauce

7 pinches of sea salt

Directions

1. Combine all ingredients in a food processor and blend until the mixture is smooth.

*Use the hummus as a dip and snack on fresh veggies.

Cucumber Bites with Tofu Spread

1 lb. organic, extra-firm tofu, drained

Handful dill

Handful scallions, chives and green onions

sea salt, to taste

1 tablespoon lemon juice

1 tablespoon white miso

3-4 cucumbers, peeled and sliced into 1/4–inch rounds

Directions

1. Combine all the ingredients except the cucumbers into a blender. Blend until creamy.

2. Arrange the cucumber slices on a plate and put a spoonful of the tofu spread on top of each cucumber slice.

Roasted Garbanzo Beans

1 can (15 ounces) organic garbanzo beans/chickpeas

1 tablespoon safflower oil

1 medium sized lime, juiced

sea salt and cayenne pepper to taste (and/or any spices of your choice)

Directions

1. Preheat oven to 450°F.

2. Drain the can of garbanzo beans and rinse.

3. In a bowl, mix the garbanzo beans with oil, lime juice, salt and cayenne pepper.

4. Spread the garbanzo beans on a baking sheet, and bake for 15 minutes on one side, then flip the garbanzo beans and bake for another 15 minutes on the other side.

*Watch carefully to avoid burning the chickpeas; you want them to be browned and crisp. If your preference is for them to be a little soft but still crunchy after flipping, just bake for 7-8 minutes on the opposite side.

Homemade Larabar Balls

½ cup walnuts

¼ cup raisins

Pinch of sea salt

Directions

1. Place all ingredients into a food processor until a sticky dough is formed.

2. Shape into balls and store in the refrigerator until ready to serve.

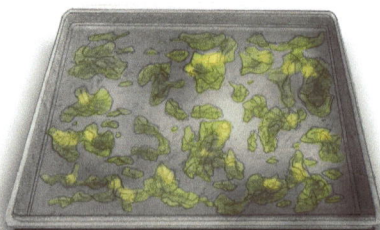

Kale Chips

1 bunch of kale

Olive oil spray

Sea salt, freshly ground pepper, garlic powder, lemon zest, and/or dill weed to taste

Directions

1. Preheat oven to 350°F.

2. Pull the kale leaves from the stem, and tear the leaves into 3-inch pieces (make sure the leaves are washed and dried).

3. Spray the sheet pan with a thin layer of olive oil and place kale leaves on the pan.

4. Spray olive oil evenly on the kale leaves, and then season the leaves with the seasonings of your choice.

5. Place in the preheated oven for 5-10 minutes or until crisp. Then serve immediately.

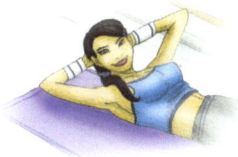

HEALTHY MIND & BODY
WORKING OUT IS FUN!

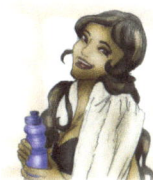

A Healthy Mind Leads to a Healthy Body

The team at FamilyDoctor.org[55] says, "Your body responds to the way you think, feel and act. This is often called the 'mind/body connection.' When you are stressed, anxious or upset, your body tries to tell you that something isn't right." Sometimes, the body communicates with the mind through subtle pains or tensions, while other times, the body can communicate through signals as serious as a heart attack. Unfortunately, many people ignore these minor signals, which can lead to the more major effects on the body, such as weight gain, disease, or malfunctions of vital organs. This is why it's important to listen to your body and to keep a healthy mind.

One of the most common ways that women deal with stress is by stress eating. This means that when anything in life seems stressful, the stressed individual seeks comfort in food. The following are some common situations in which one might reach for food to comfort him- or herself. See if you can relate to any of these:

- You've had a bad day at work, and the first thing you do when you come home is open the pantry.

- The kids are getting on your nerves, and you "treat" both them and yourself to some easy fast food.

- Your car breaks down, and the first thing you think to do, once convenient of course, is to track down a candy bar.

- You've got an endless to-do list, and food is always the first thing on your mind, whenever you get five minutes in between tasks.

- It's time to give yourself a quick break, and a pre-packaged snack seems like an extremely convenient form of satisfaction.

Stress eating is harmful to your body, because you eat both unwanted and empty calories all at once. In addition, your self-esteem and confidence can plummet. With a regular workout regiment and a clean diet, your self-esteem and confidence are *boosted*, along with your energy levels and self-image.

With a powerful mind, you will empower your body and vise versa. It's up to you to gain control over you mind so that you can listen when your body sends you signals that something is wrong. The best way to empower your mind and listen to your body is by quieting the mind. Just as you have conversations with others, your body has conversations with the mind, in which there alternates a speaker and a listener. Quiet the speaker in the mind and allow it time to be the listener. Through yoga and/or meditation, the mind and body may conduct a more recognizable conversation, in which you can clearly recognize the wishes of your body.

Perhaps you've been receiving messages that dairy doesn't suit your body well. Maybe your body is trying to tell you that it's had enough of processed foods, or maybe it's trying to tell you that it wants to cut down on meat consumption. The next time you have a nagging feeling that your body wants to communicate important information to you, do yourself and your body a favor. Stop, sit down, close your eyes, and listen.

When meditating and when doing yoga, the most important component is the breath. When you concentrate on the breath, the mind quiets more easily, and the muscles and organs in your body function in a way that allows them to communicate more easily. Don't be upset at yourself for having passing thoughts—it's bound to happen, and it's okay that it does. As one thought passes, visualize yourself picking that thought up with your fingers and putting it into a box. This will help separate your thoughts from your mind, giving your mind room to breathe and de-clutter.

Remember, what you tell your inner self reflects upon the outer self. If you find yourself being held back by a negative self-image or a negative outlook, your chances of losing weight are far less. Give yourself a 30-day meditation challenge, and you will be surprised with your results. *Everyone* can gain something from clearing and cleansing the mind and body.

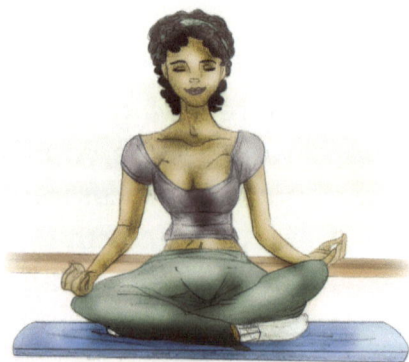

AFTERWORD

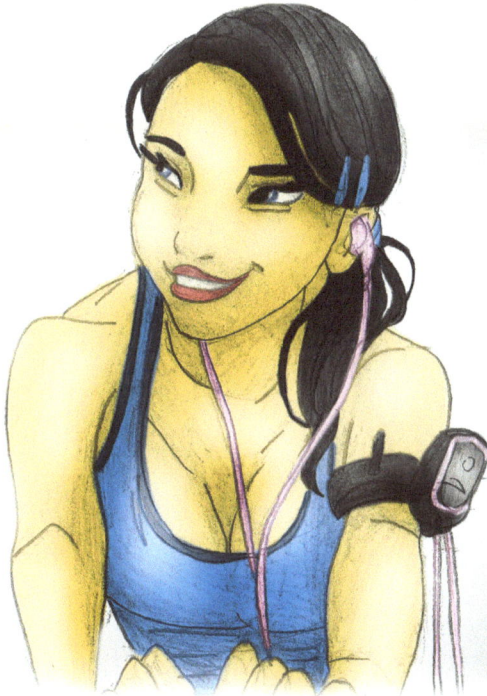

NOW THAT YOU ARE EQUIPPED WITH all the tools you need to be successful, it's time to keep moving forward. This is a journey that will continue throughout your life, and the rewards will just keep getting better and better! Give yourself the gift of health and wellness, because this is the gift that keeps on giving. Just remember the tips you've learned here, and you'll do great! And if you can't remember absolutely everything, *Click it to Rip it* will always be here to remind you of anything you may have forgotten. So, just in case you didn't remember, you are *amazing*, and you are worth it! By making healthy decisions one day at a time, you will wake up one morning and find yourself in the midst of living and embracing a healthy lifestyle. Changing your lifestyle is a great accomplishment, and you should be proud of yourself! Now, go on with your beautiful new self! Give yourself the health and happiness you deserve!

RESOURCES

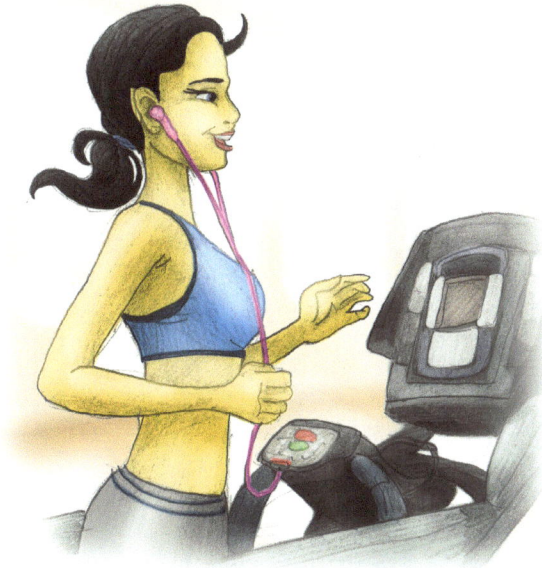

BELOW ARE RESOURCES FOR YOU to use in your quest to *Click it to Rip it*. The resources below are a tiny snippet of the wealth of information that is available. Speak to your doctor and nutritionist, because they'll have resources for you too.

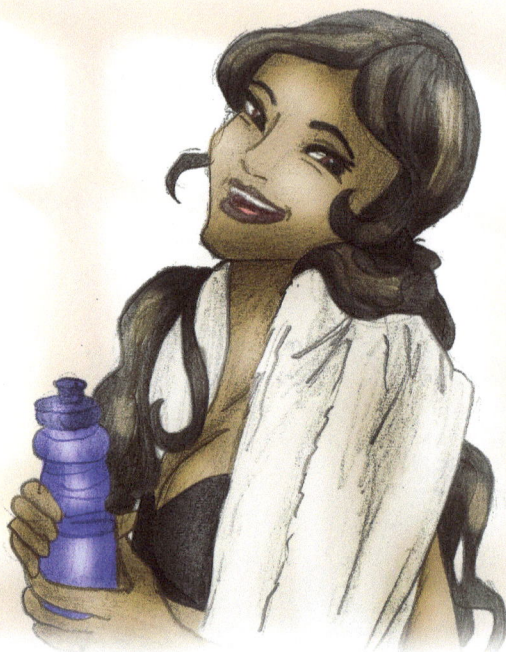

General Health and Fitness Websites

WebMD.com

Healthandfitnessohio.com

Prevention.com

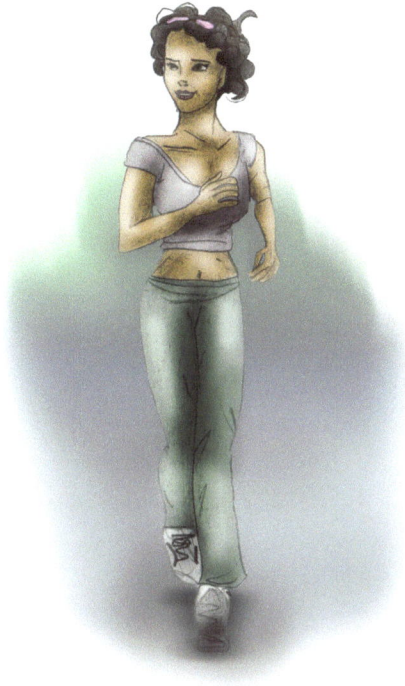

Restaurant Guides

Healthydiningfinder.com/home

Cleanplates.com

Heart.org

Eatwellguide.org

Happycow.net

CLICK IT TO RIP IT

Supplement Websites

ChampionNutrition.com

Gardenoflife.com

GNC.com

Weight Loss Support Groups

Weightlossbuddy.com

Facebook.com/GirlfriendsWeightLossSupportGroup

Sparkpeople.com

Extrapounds.com

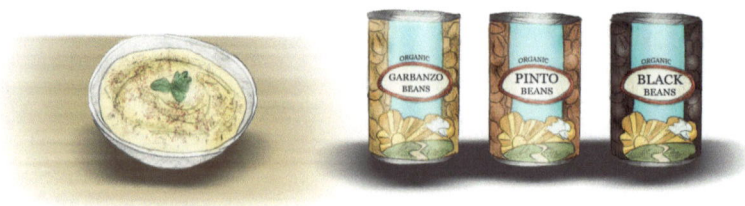

Cookbooks

The EatingWell Healthy in a Hurry Cookbook: 150 Delicious Recipes for Simple, Everyday Suppers in 45 Minutes or Less, Jim Romanoff, The Editors of EatingWell

RESOURCES

The America's Test Kitchen Healthy Family Cookbook: A New, Healthier Way to Cook Everything from America's Most Trusted Test Kitchen, America's Test Kitchen

Cooking Light Fresh Food Fast: Weeknight Meals: Over 280 Incredible Supper Solutions, Editors of Cooking Light Magazine

Eat to Lose, Eat to Win: Your Grab-n-Go Action Plan for a Slimmer, Healthier You, Rachel Beller, MS, RD

Diabetes and Heart Healthy Cookbook, American Diabetes Association, American Heart Association

The Diabetic Gourmet Cookbook: More Than 200 Healthy Recipes from Homestyle Favorites to Restaurant Classics, Editors of Diabetic Gourmet Magazine

Vegetarian, Alice Hart

My Sweet Vegan: passionate about dessert, Hannah Kaminsky

Veganomicon: The Ultimate Vegan Cookbook, Isa Chandra Moskowitz and Terry Hope Romero

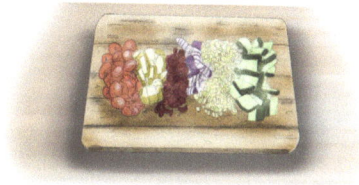

Pure Vegan: 70 Recipes for Beautiful Meals and Clean Living, Joseph Shuldiner

Vegan Yum Yum: Decadent (But Doable) Animal-Free Recipes for Entertaining and Everyday, Lauren Ulm

Blogs | Magazines

Eatingwell.com

Cookinglight.com

Shape.com

Fitnessglo.com

Womenshealthmag.com

Fitnessmagazine.com

Health.com

Self.com

Cleaneatingmag.com

SOURCES CITED

"4 Health Side Effects of Diet Soda," accessed April 29, 2013 http://www.fitday.com/fitness-articles/nutrition/healthy-eating/4-health-side-effects-of-diet-soda.html#b

"6 Health Benefits of Dark Chocolate," Fit Today, accessed April 23, 2013, http://www.fitday.com/fitness-articles/nutrition/healthy-eating/6-health-benefits-of-dark-chocolate.html

"6 Different Types of Exercise Mats." Fit Today, accessed March 4, 2013 http://www.fitday.com/fitness-articles/fitness/equipment/6-different-types-of-exercise-mats.html#b

"Mind/Body Connection: How Your Emotions Affect Your Health," accessed July 21, 2013, http://familydoctor.org/familydoctor/en/prevention-wellness/emotional-wellbeing/mental-health/mind-body-connection-how-your-emotions-affect-your- health.html

Bumgardner, Wendy. "Heart Rate Zones." About.com Guide, Updated April 01, 2012; accessed March 26,

2013, http://walking.about.com/cs/fitnesswalking/a/
hearttraining_2.htm

Charlebois, Derek B.S. CPT and Katie Lobliner. "Women's
Body Bible: Training, Diet & Supplementation!" accessed Feb. 21, 2013, http://www.muscleandstrength.
com/articles/womens-body-bible.html

Clark, Shannon. "The Top 10 Reasons to Use Full Body
Workouts." accessed Feb. 11, 2013, http://www.
bodybuilding.com/fun/top-10-full-body-workout-
benefits.htm

Davis, Brenna, "What Do Women Wear to Work Out?" Demand
Media; accessed March 5, 2013, http://healthyliving.
azcentral.com/women-wear-work-out-3901.html

Douban, Gigi, "Your Gym's Dirty Little Secrets," *Women's
Health*; accessed March 1, 2013, http://healthyliving.
msn.com/fitness/your-gyms-dirty-little-secrets

Fonooni, Neghar. http://www.negharfonooni.com.

Fonooni, Neghar. "Teach Your Female Personal Training
Clients to Train Like Men." August 9, 2011; accessed
Feb. 26, 2013, http://www.theptdc.com/2011/08/
teach-your-female-personal-training-clients-to-train-
like-men/

Glanville, Nicole, PTI REP Level 3. "Heart Rate Monitors
Review." accessed March 7, 2013, http://www.

weightlossresources.co.uk/exercise/reviews/heart-rate-monitor.htm.

Grossner, Colleen, Registered Dietitian. http://fresh-you.blogspot.com/.

Harmon, Jane. "What are resistance bands?" Edited By: Niki Foster; accessed March 5, 2013, http://www.wisegeek.com/what-are-resistance-bands.htm

Hatfield, Frederick C. (n.d.). "Bodybuilding According to Joe Weider." accessed Feb. 10, 2013, http://www.bodybuilding.com/fun/drsquat3.htm

Holland, Tom and Megan McMorris. *Beat the Gym: Personal Trainer Secrets--Without the Personal Trainer Price Tag*. New York: William Morrow, an imprint of HarperCollins Publishers, 2011.

Hyman, Mark, MD, Practicing physician. "How Diet Soda Makes You Fat (and Other Food and Diet Industry Secrets)." accessed April 29, 2013, http://www.huffingtonpost.com/dr-mark-hyman/diet-soda-health_b_2698494.html

Jegtvig, Shereen. "Weight Management: How Many Calories You Need Per Day." About.com Guide, Updated March 13, 2013; accessed April 18, 2013, http://nutrition.about.com/od/changeyourdiet/a/calguide.htm.

Major, Kenneth J, *The Pre-Industrial Sources of Power: Muscle Power,* History Today Volume: 30 Issue: 3 1980; accessed March 5, 2013, http://www.history today.com/j-kenneth-major/pre-industrial-sources-power-muscle-power

Mayo Clinic staff. "Exercise: 7 benefits of regular physical activity." accessed March 11, 2013, http://www. mayoclinic.com/health/exercise/HQ01676.

Morris, Desmond. *The Naked Woman: A Study of the Female Body.* New York: Thomas DunneBooks. St. Martin's Press, 2004; accessed Feb. 13, 2013, pages 5, 117, 118. From THE NAKED WOMEN © 2005 by Desmond Morris. Reprinted by permission of St. Martin's Press. All rights reserved. http://books. google.com/books?id=Wa9zntiEKeAC&pg=PA117&source=gbs_toc_r&cad=4#v=onepage&q&f=false

Nelson, Rachel. "Medicine Ball Training Information." Nov 22, 2009; accessed March 6, 2013, http://www. livestrong.com/article/38753-medicine-ball-training-information/#ixzz2MnJLdLle

Pikul, Corrie. "13 Things Every Woman Doesn't Know About Her Own Body." accessed Feb. 13,2013, http://www.oprah.com/health/Womens-Health-Triva-Fascinating-Facts-About-Womens-Bodies/3#ixzz2Kmvr6hnQ

SOURCES CITED

Presley, Susan. "Resistance Band Guide." Demand Media; accessed March 6, 2013, http://healthyliving.azcentral. com/resistance-band-guide-7511.html.

Rail, Kevin. "Flat Bench Workouts" June 4, 2010; accessed March 6, 2013, http://www.livestrong.com/article/ article/139178-flat-bench-workouts/#ixzz2MnHdFAka

Reed, Bill. "Saved by the kettlebell: Bored with the same old gym routine? Try working out the Russian way." *Winnipeg Free Press: Print Edition,* Fitness Trends, May 9, 2009; accessed March 4, 2013, http://www. winnipegfreepress.com/arts-and-life/life/health/ saved-by-the-kettlebell-44633867.html

Sarnataro, Barbara Russi. "Fitness Basics: The Exercise Bike Is Back: It's time for another look at an old fitness favorite." Reviewed by Louise Chang, MD; accessed March 6, 2013, http://www.webmd.com/fitness-exercise/ features/fitness-basics-exercise-bike-is-back

Steen, Darin L. and Dr. Mercola. "Personal Trainer Says: Most People are Wasting Their Time Working Out." October 5, 2010; accessed Feb. 26, 2013, http://fitness. mercola.com/sites/fitness/archive/2010/10/05/dont-make-these-mistakes-with-your-workouts.aspx

The Original Swiss Ball. accessed March 6, 2013, http:// www.swissballs.com/

Turcotte, Michele MS, RD. "The Effects of Exercise on Serotonin Levels." Apr. 26, 2011; accessed March 11, 2013, http://www.livestrong.com/article/22590-effects-exercise-serotonin-levels/.

Yale School of Medicine. "Using Free Weights for Resistance Training." Yale Medical Group.com, accessed March 6, 2013, http://www.yalemedicalgroup.org/stw/Page.asp?PageID=STW046092

"YOUR TARGET HEART RATE," accessed March 11, 2013; http://www.thewalkingsite.com/thr.html

Waehner, Paige. "Before You Buy a Heart Rate Monitor." About.com Guide, updated April 22, 2009; accessed March 7, 2013, http://exercise.about.com/cs/exercisegear/bb/byb_HRM.htm

Waehner, Paige. "The BOSU Ball: Enhance your balance and strength." About.com Guide, updated July 15, 2011; accessed March 6, 2013, http://exercise.about.com/cs/exercisegear/a/bosu.htm

WebMD Medical Reference. "Protein shakes." Reviewed by Kimball Johnson, MD on June 23, 2012, accessed April 18, 2013, http://www.webmd.com/diet/protein-shakes

Williamson, Marianne. A *Return to Love: Reflections on the Principles of A Course in Miracles*.New York: HarperCollins, 1992.

END NOTES

[1] Click it to Rip it is to be a registered trademarked by Anna Petras.

[2] Shannon Clark, "The Top 10 Reasons to Use a Fully Body Workout," accessed Feb. 11, 2013, www.bodybuilding.com/fun/top-10-full-body-workout-benefits.htm.

[3] Clark, www.bodybuilding.com/fun/top-10-full-body-workout-benefits.htm.

[4] Turcotte, Michele MS, RD, "The Effects of Exercise on Serotonin Levels," Apr. 26, 2011, accessed March 11, 2013, http://www.livestrong.com/article/22590-effects-exercise-serotonin-levels/.

[5] Mayo Clinic staff, "Exercise: 7 benefits of regular physical activity," accessed March 11, 2013, http://www.mayoclinic.com/health/exercise/HQ01676.

[6] Mayo Clinic staff, "Exercise: 7 benefits of regular physical activity," accessed March 11, 2013, http://www.mayoclinic.com/health/exercise/HQ01676.

[7] "YOUR TARGET HEART RATE," accessed March 11, 2013; http://www.thewalkingsite.com/thr.html.

[8] Waehner, Paige, "Before You Buy a Heart Rate Monitor," About.com Guide, updated April 22, 2009, accessed March 7, 2013, http://exercise.about.com/cs/exercisegear/bb/byb_HRM.htm.

[9] Glanville, Nicole, PTI REP Level 3, "Heart Rate Monitors Review," accessed March 7, 2013, http://www.weightlossresources.co.uk/exercise/reviews/heart-rate-monitor.htm.

[10] Glanville, "Heart Rate Monitors Review," accessed March 7, 2013, http://www.weightlossresources.co.uk/exercise/reviews/heart-rate-monitor.htm.

[11] Bumgardner, Wendy, "Heart Rate Zones," About.com Guide, Updated April 01, 2012; accessed March 26, 2013, http://walking.about.com/cs/fitnesswalking/a/hearttraining_2.htm.

[12] "YOUR TARGET HEART RATE," accessed March 11, 2013; http://www.thewalkingsite.com/thr.html.

[13] Bumgardner, "Heart Rate Zones," About.com Guide, Updated April 01, 2012; accessed March 26, 2013, http://walking.about.com/cs/fitnesswalking/a/hearttraining_2.htm.

[14] "YOUR TARGET HEART RATE," accessed March 11, 2013; http://www.thewalkingsite.com/thr.html.

[15] "YOUR TARGET HEART RATE," accessed March 11, 2013; http://www.thewalkingsite.com/thr.html.

[16] Bumgardner, "Heart Rate Zones," About.com Guide, Updated April 01, 2012; accessed March 26, 2013, http://walking.about.com/cs/fitnesswalking/a/hearttraining_2.htm.

[17] Grossner, Colleen, Registered Dietitian, http://fresh-you.blogspot.com/.

[18] Pikul, http://www.oprah.com/health/Womens-Health-Triva-Fascinating-Facts-About- Womens-Bodies/3#ixzz2Kmvr6hnQ.

[19] From THE NAKED WOMEN © 2005 by Desmond Morris. Reprinted by permission of St. Martin's Press. All rights reserved. http://www.amazon.com/Naked-Woman-Study-Female-Body/dp/0312338538#reader_0312338538, 5.

[20] From THE NAKED WOMEN © 2005 by Desmond Morris. Reprinted by permission of St. Martin's Press. All rights reserved. http://books.google.com/books?id=Wa9zntiEKeAC&pg=PA117&source=gbs_toc_r&cad=4#v=onepage&q&f=false, 118.

21 From *THE NAKED WOMEN* © 2005 by Desmond Morris. Reprinted by permission of St. Martin's Press. All rights reserved. http://books.google.com/books?id=Wa9zntiEKeAC&pg=PA117&source=gbs_toc_r&cad=4#v=onepage&q&f=false, 117.

22 Corrie Pikul, "13 Things Every Woman Doesn't Know About Her Own Body," accessed Feb. 13, 2013, http://www.oprah.com/health/Womens-Health-Triva-Fascinating-Facts-About-Womens-Bodies/3#ixzz2Kmvr6hnQ.

23 Pikul, http://www.oprah.com/health/Womens-Health-Triva-Fascinating-Facts-About- Womens-Bodies/3#ixzz2Kmvr6hnQ.

24 Charlebois, Derek B.S. CPT and Katie Lobliner, "Women's Body Bible: Training, Diet & Supplementation!" accessed Feb. 21, 2013, http://www.muscleandstrength.com/articles/womens-body-bible.html.

25 Charlebois, Derek B.S. CPT and Katie Lobliner. http://www.muscleandstrength.com/articles/womens-body-bible.html.

26 Steen, Darin L. and Dr. Mercola, "Personal Trainer Says: Most People are Wasting Their Time Working Out," accessed Feb. 26, 2013, http://fitness.mercola.com/sites/fitness/archive/2010/10/05/dont-make-these-mistakes-with-your-workouts.aspx.

27 Holland, Tom and Megan McMorris, *Beat the Gym: Personal Trainer Secrets--Without the Personal Trainer Price Tag*, New York: William Morrow, an imprint of HarperCollins Publishers, 2011, 3.

28 Fonooni, "Teach Your Female Personal Training Clients to Train Like Men," accessed Feb. 26, 2013, http://www.theptdc.com/2011/08/teach-your-female-personal-training-clients-to-train-like-men.

29 Douban, Gigi, "Your Gym's Dirty Little Secrets," accessed March 1, 2013, http://healthyliving.msn.com/fitness/your-gyms-dirty-little-secrets, Women's Health.

30 Yale School of Medicine. "Using Free Weights for Resistance Training." Yale Medical Group.com, accessed March 6, 2013, http://www.yalemedicalgroup.org/stw/Page.asp?PageID=STW046092.

31 Yale School of Medicine. "Using Free Weights for Resistance Training." Yale Medical Group.com, accessed March 6, 2013, http://www.yalemedicalgroup.org/stw/Page.asp?PageID=STW046092.

32 The Original Swiss Ball, accessed March 6, 2013, http://www.swissballs.com/.

33 Reed, Bill, "Saved by the kettlebell: Bored with the same old gym routine? Try working out the Russian way," *Winnipeg Free Press: Print Edition*, Fitness Trends, May 9, 2009. accessed March 4, 2013, http://www.winnipegfreepress.com/arts-and-life/life/health/saved-by-the-kettlebell-44633867.html.

34 Harmon, Jane, "What are resistance bands?" accessed March 5, 2013, Edited By: Niki Foster http://www.wisegeek.com/what-are-resistance-bands.htm.

35 Presley, Susan, "Resistance Band Guide," Demand Media; accessed March 6, 2013, http://healthyliving.azcentral.com/resistance-band-guide-7511.html.

36 Rail, Kevin, "Flat Bench Workouts," June 4, 2010; accessed March 6, 2013, http://www.livestrong.com/article/article/139178-flat-bench-workouts/#ixzz2MnHdFAka.

37 Waehner, Paige, "The BOSU Ball: Enhance your balance and strength," About.com Guide, updated July 15, 2011, accessed March 6, 2013, http://exercise.about.com/cs/exercisegear/a/bosu.htm.

38 Nelson, Rachel, "Medicine Ball Training Information," Nov 22, 2009; accessed March 6, 2013, http://www.livestrong.com/article/38753-medicine-ball-training-information/#ixzz2MnJLdLIe.

END NOTES

[39] "6 Different Types of Exercise Mats," Fit Today, accessed March 4, 2013, http://www.fitday.com/fitness-articles/fitness/equipment/6-different-types-of-exercise-mats.html#b.

[40] "6 Different Types of Exercise Mats," Fit Today, accessed March 4, 2013, http://www.fitday.com/fitness-articles/fitness/equipment/6-different-types-of-exercise-mats.html#b.

[41] "6 Different Types of Exercise Mats," Fit Today, accessed March 4, 2013, http://www.fitday.com/fitness-articles/fitness/equipment/6-different-types-of-exercise-mats.html#b.

[42] "6 Different Types of Exercise Mats," Fit Today, accessed March 4, 2013, http://www.fitday.com/fitness-articles/fitness/equipment/6-different-types-of-exercise-mats.html#b.

[43] Major, Kenneth J, *The Pre-Industrial Sources of Power: Muscle Power*, History Today Volume: 30 Issue: 3 1980, accessed March 5, 2013, http://www.historytoday.com/j-kenneth-major/pre-industrial-sources-power-muscle-power.

[44] Sarnataro, Barbara Russi, "Fitness Basics: The Exercise Bike Is Back: It's time for another look at an old fitness favorite," Reviewed by Louise Chang, MD, accessed March 6, 2013, http://www.webmd.com/fitness-exercise/features/fitness-basics-exercise-bike-is-back.

[45] Davis, "What Do Women Wear to Work Out?" accessed March 5, 2013, Demand Media, http://healthyliving.azcentral.com/women-wear-work-out-3901.html.

[46] Davis, "What Do Women Wear to Work Out?" accessed March 5, 2013, Demand Media, http://healthyliving.azcentral.com/women-wear-work-out-3901.html.

[47] Davis, "What Do Women Wear to Work Out?" accessed March 5, 2013, Demand Media, http://healthyliving.azcentral.com/women-wear-work-out-3901.html.

[48] Tracy, Nancy, "Color Psychology and Dieting: How Different Colors Affect Your Appetite: Shed Pounds with Strategic Use of Color," Yahoo! Contributor Network, Dec 7, 2009, accessed March 19, 2013, http://voices.yahoo.com/color-psychology-dieting-different-colors-4973404.html.

[49] WebMD Medical Reference, "Protein shakes," Reviewed by Kimball Johnson, MD on June 23, 2012, accessed April 18, 2013, http://www.webmd.com/diet/protein-shakes.

[50] Jegtvig, Shereen, "Weight Management: How Many Calories You Need Per Day," About.com Guide, Updated March 13, 2013, accessed April 18, 2013, http://nutrition.about.com/od/changeyourdiet/a/calguide.htm.

[51] Shereen, "Weight Management: How Many Calories You Need Per Day," About.com Guide, Updated March 13, 2013, accessed April 18, 2013, http://nutrition.about.com/od/changeyourdiet/a/calguide.htm.

[52] Hyman, Mark, MD, Practicing physician, "How Diet Soda Makes You Fat (and Other Food and Diet Industry Secrets)," accessed April 29, 2013, http://www.huffingtonpost.com/dr-mark-hyman/diet-soda-health_b_2698494.html.

[53] "4 Health Side Effects of Diet Soda," accessed April 29, 2013 http://www.fitday.com/fitness-articles/nutrition/healthy-eating/4-health-side-effects-of-diet-soda.html#b.

[54] "6 Health Benefits of Dark Chocolate," Fit Today, accessed April 23, 2013, http://www.fitday.com/fitness-articles/nutrition/healthy-eating/6-health-benefits-of- dark-chocolate.html#b.

[55] "Mind/Body Connection: How Your Emotions Affect Your Health," accessed July 21, 2013, http://familydoctor.org/familydoctor/en/prevention-wellness/emotional- wellbeing/mental-health/mind-body-connection-how-your-emotions-affect-your-health.html

www.ingramcontent.com/pod-product-compliance
Lightning Source LLC
Chambersburg PA
CBHW040129270326
41928CB00001B/1